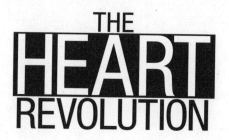

THE
HEART
REVOLUTION

THE HEART REVOLUTION

The B Vitamin Breakthrough that Lowers Homocysteine, Cuts Your Risk of Heart Disease, and Protects Your Health

Kilmer McCully, M.D.
and Martha McCully

HarperCollins*Publishers*

This book is not intended to replace medical advice or to be a substitute for a physician. Always seek the advice of a physician before beginning any diet and/or exercise program.

HarperCollins books may be purchased for educational, business, or sales promotional use. For information please write: Special Markets Department, HarperCollins Publishers, Inc., 10 East 53rd Street, New York, NY 10022.

FIRST EDITION

Designed by Liane Fuji

ISBN 0-06-019237-2

99 00 01 02 03 ❖/RRD 10 9 8 7 6 5 4 3 2 1

To Nina
for making the Heart Revolution possible

Contents

Acknowledgments

My discovery of the association between homocysteine and arteriosclerosis in 1968 was aided by my colleagues of the Human Genetics Unit of the Massachusetts General Hospital. In 1965 pediatricians Vivian Shih and Mary Efron traced and identified the index case of homocystinuria in the medical literature, as first published in the New England Journal of Medicine in 1933. They were able to identify this first case because the mother of their patient, a nine-year-old girl with homocystinuria, told them about the girl's uncle who had died of a similar disease over thirty years before. I thank Vivian Shih and Harvey Levy for encouraging my interest in the vascular pathology of homocystinuria and for sharing their findings prior to publication of another important case. This second case was a two-month-old boy with homocystinuria and cystathioninuria who was the index case of cobalamin C disease in the medical literature. Comparison of this second critically important case with the findings in the case from 1933 made possible the conclusion that homocysteine causes arteriosclerosis by damaging the cells and tissues of the arteries. I also thank John Littlefield, whose encouragement and interest further aided my understanding of the significance of this discovery.

Although I never met the great biochemist Vincent Du-Vigneaud, I wish to acknowledge his discovery of homocysteine in 1932 and his subsequent pioneering work on the importance of this amino acid in biochemistry and nutrition. I also thank Giulio Cantoni and Harvey Mudd, who introduced me to the biochemistry of homocysteine and methionine during my two years in their laboratory at the National Institutes of Health in Bethesda, Maryland, in 1960. Without the pioneering discoveries of these outstanding biochemists, a fundamental understanding of the cause of the disease homocystinuria would not have been available before I first examined these two unique cases in 1968.

During my pathology residency and years as a staff pathologist at Massachusetts General Hospital, my interest and knowledge of the pathology of arteriosclerosis were especially aided by Benjamin Castleman, Robert Scully, and James Caulfield. I acknowledge these colleagues for their support and encouragement in the several years immediately following my discovery of the association between homocysteine and arteriosclerosis.

I also thank Moses Suzman of South Africa, whose knowledge of arteriosclerosis and cardiology helped me to understand the importance of homocysteine in the history of arteriosclerosis research. He was a colleague of James Rinehart of Berkeley, California, who discovered that dietary deficiency of vitamin B6 causes arteriosclerosis in monkeys. Suzman also aided my understanding of how the investigations of Ignatowsky, Anitschkow, and Newburgh helped to establish the nutritional origin of arteriosclerosis.

I thank Guido Pontecorvo, the founder of the Genetics Department of Glasgow University, Scotland, for introducing me to the principles of classical and molecular genetics. Without his guidance and encouragement, I would not have been able to develop my unique approach to understanding the pathology of inherited diseases, especially homocystinuria. I also thank James Watson for his guidance and for his patience with me during my several months in his laboratory at Harvard.

During my student years, several prominent medical scientists and teachers encouraged my interest in medical research. I especially thank Konrad Bloch for introducing me to the biochemistry of cholesterol in his biochemistry course at Harvard and for stimulating my interest and excitement about biochemistry research during my several months as a research assistant in his laboratory. I thank Paul Zamecnik and Lewis Engel for their patient guidance of my interest in medical research during my student and fellowship years at Harvard Medical School and Massachusetts General Hospital. I thank Louis Fieser for his masterful introduction to the organic chemistry of polycyclic hydrocarbons and cholesterol and for the opportunity to participate in his research study of the purification of cholesterol in his laboratory at Harvard. I also gratefully acknowledge the wonderful experience of learning with the superb scientists B. F. Skinner at Harvard and James Bonner at California Institute of Technology.

In the 1970s Edward Gruberg and Stephen Raymond of Massachusetts Institute of Technology became interested in the homocysteine theory of heart disease and published the first book on the subject in 1981 entitled *Beyond Cholesterol*. I thank them for their perseverance, persistence, and clear exposition of the scientific evidence before human clinical and epidemiological studies proved the validity of the theory in the 1980s and 1990s.

During the 1970s and 1980s, my scientific collaborators Roberta Ricci of Rome, Italy; Pierre Clopath of Zurich, Switzerland; Andrzej Olszewski of Warsaw, Poland; Marek Naruszewicz of Sczczin, Poland; and Michael Vezeridis of the Providence (Rhode Island) V.A. Medical Center were of invaluable assistance in developing scientific evidence to support the homocysteine theory. I thank them, and I also thank the students, technologists, and assistants who faithfully and enthusiastically assisted in my scientific laboratory investigations. I also thank F. William Sunderman, Jr., of the University of Connecticut Health Center for his friendship and professional encouragement during difficult years.

Finally, I thank my devoted wife, Annina Elena McCully, for her steadfast and resolute faith in my scientific work. The homocysteine revolution could not have become a reality without her companionship throughout the past forty-three years.

We offer a special thank you to Amanda Urban for making this book possible and to Megan Newman for her skillful and intelligent editing of the manuscript.

Foreword

Kilmer McCully's tale is as old as history. On a grand scale, it's the story of Galileo. Startling, revolutionary ideas have always faced an uphill battle, and particularly in science and medicine. The burden of proof, the finality of fact, rests heavily on the scientist, especially when lives may be at stake. And on a less academic level, people resist change. They don't like having to rethink their assumptions.

One assumption was still prevalent when I became aware of Kilmer McCully: High levels of blood cholesterol, often presumably caused by a high intake of dietary cholesterol in the form of meats and fats, was considered a key factor in heart disease. The correlary of this assumption was that lowering blood cholesterol would lower the risk of heart disease. Cholesterol was seen as a crucial marker for heart disease risk, and high blood cholesterol was—and still is—often treated with drugs in an effort to bring it to within "normal" limits.

A lot of money had been funneled into studying cholesterol, and a sizable number of scientists had based their careers upon it. When Kilmer McCully began publishing his research on homocysteine in the 1970s—research that suggested a new pathway for the genesis of heart disease, a pathway that relegated cholesterol firmly to a secondary position—several government agencies were in the thick of gearing up for a major public-health directive about cholesterol. Their goal: to make cholesterol a household word. They succeeded so successfully that today's supermarkets and food advertisements are plastered with "No Cholesterol" claims, used as a synonym for "healthy." If there's anything that the average citizen has now absorbed about heart disease, it's that cholesterol levels should be checked and that cholesterol in foods should be avoided at all costs.

To say that McCully's ideas were unwelcome at the cholesterol feast in the late 1970s would be a mammoth understatement. Many people had invested heavily in the cholesterol theory, and few wanted to hear it challenged. And, on a more benign level, there just wasn't interest in new ideas when the connection to cholesterol looked so exciting and promising— why clutter the field with obscure new theories? But what happened then, in McCully's life, was not benign. This was what convinced me in 1997 to write an article about his experience for the *New York Times Magazine*. In short order, McCully lost his grant support and with it his appointments at Harvard and Massachusetts General Hospital. He was told by the director of

Mass General that it was felt at Harvard that he had not proved his theory, and another official of the hospital told him not to promulgate his ideas to the press; he didn't want the names of Harvard and Mass General associated with the homocysteine theory.

The process of losing the position that had defined his life took a year and a half, during which McCully's life was over-shadowed by a steady and humiliating march toward jobless-ness. Back in 1970 McCully's research on homocysteine and arteriosclerosis had been praised by a special Scientific Advisory Committee at Mass General as an illustration of "the un-predictable, important contributions which can come when an imaginative, skilled worker is given free rein to follow his ideas and findings"; by 1977, with the pathology department under a new chairman, McCully's laboratory at Mass General was taken away, and he lost staff support for his research. Two months later, he was confronted with an academic Catch–22: He was informed that his appointment at Mass General would not be renewed in 1979 and that unless he could ob-tain another NIH grant his salary would be reduced to almost nothing by January 1978. Under those conditions, with no position or laboratory, it became almost impossible to obtain further grant support. After a series of mortifying meetings with top people at Mass General and Harvard, during which his requests for more time were denied, McCully finally found himself—at mid-career, with two children in college—looking for a new job. That job was a long time in coming.

For two unnerving years, McCully—with his pedigree of a Harvard College degree, Harvard Medical School degree, and fourteen years professorship at Harvard—could not get past a first interview anywhere in the country. Between 1979 and

1981 he made fifty-one contacts with potential employers, from San Diego to Dallas to Connecticut, and each one evaporated. He was repeatedly advised to give up his research—the ambition that had defined his life since boyhood—and accept a lower-level staff position as a pathologist. Then McCully began to hear rumors of "poison" phone calls from Harvard, of unflattering comments about his habits, his work, his character. Only when he took steps toward engaging a prominent Boston lawyer to represent him in a case against officials of Mass General and Harvard did a firm job offer finally come through, at a much less prominent institution, the V.A. Hospital in Providence, Rhode Island, where he still works today.

It was clear that McCully's life and career had been seriously damaged by his pursuit of the homocysteine theory. Why was he made such a pariah? The most obvious answer is the one mentioned above: that the cholesterol bandwagon was loaded up and ready to go, and nobody involved wanted to change direction. But that answer itself raises further, and disturbing, questions. Is the scientific system set up in such a way to encourage following the idea of the moment? Is there a tendency toward scientific tunnel vision that is somehow intensified by the ways in which research is conducted and funded? Who exactly was it who had so much to lose if cholesterol took a back seat?

Many scientists feel, McCully among them, that our current research system does indeed reward accepted ideas. Science has become a team endeavor, and working by committee often discourages individual dissent. Team members can easily become swept up in the general enthusiasm toward a particular approach, and it becomes difficult to change direction or even to perceive weak spots in one's logic or results. Research has also become Big Science, with each new project entailing large outlays of resources, further discouraging the tinkering and serendipity that can lead to breakthroughs or new directions.

Finally, there is the problem of who's making the money, and in this case, it has been the drug companies that manufacture cholesterol-lowering therapies. The antidote to homocysteine, in McCully's model, is not only simple, it's inexpensive: Eat foods rich in B vitamins, and if you like, take a multivitamin just to be sure. There are no remedies that drug manufacturers can patent and market exclusively. That's why the homocysteine theory does not attract any of the millions of corporate research dollars floating around in search of a product, and why certain manufacturers have a vested interest in keeping cholesterol, and its expensive drug treatments, in the forefront of cardiac treatment. As many scientists have pointed out, regarding not only heart disease but cancer as well, money is earned not in prevention but in treatment—with surgery, drugs, and other medical services. If you "follow the money" in medical research you arrive not at public-health advice like "eat your vegetables," but at profit-heavy interventions to treat advanced disease.

The personal toll on Kilmer McCully and his family was great, but in the 1990s his time came again—to stay. Other researchers were slowly beginning to confirm McCully's ideas, researchers working for the most part out of the reach of American science, in Sweden, Norway, the Netherlands, and Ireland. Several American scientists then became interested, and homocysteine had its breakthrough into the mainstream. Two big-name and impressive ongoing research groups, the

Physicians Health Study (a continuing survey of almost 15,000 doctors) and the Framingham Study (which has documented the population of Framingham, Massachusetts, for nearly fifty years), turned up a strong correlation between high homocysteine levels and heart-disease incidence. Articles about those correlations appeared in the two top establishment medical journals, *The New England Journal of Medicine* and the *Journal of the American Medical Association*, and each one began by citing McCully's original 1969 article on homocysteine and arteriosclerosis. In 1995, the first International Conference on Homocysteine Metabolism was held, in County Clare, Ireland, and McCully was introduced as "the father of homocysteine." That same year, McCully appeared on the *NBC Nightly News*, in a segment on homocysteine as a new risk factor for heart disease, to discuss his work and the ups and downs of his career.

The hitherto obscure word "homocysteine" was beginning to make its way into the national forum. By the time I started speaking with McCully for my *New York Times Magazine* article in 1997, ads for multivitamins were mentioning homocysteine as "an emerging risk factor for heart disease," and *Newsweek* was gearing up for a major story that featured homocysteine as one of the new "hidden causes of heart attacks." *Time* magazine ran an article headlined "Beyond Cholesterol" that told the homocysteine story and mentioned McCully as the first to make the homocysteine–heart disease connection. Now, almost two years later, many doctors routinely advise patients to take a daily multivitamin specifically to maintain high levels of B vitamins to help avert heart disease. If *homocysteine* is not yet the household word that *cholesterol* is, despite the now-persuasive evidence, it may be partially because of the problem of profits: There is no expensive prescription-drug antidote to homocysteine that would earn millions for a pharmaceutical firm, simply a fresh-foods-and-vitamins approach that anyone can follow.

Through all the painful fluctuations of his career, and that of his career discovery, homocysteine, McCully retained his drive, his equilibrium, and, perhaps most important, his sense of humor. When we retraced his work together in 1997, he acknowledged that he knows this is the way science often works: One person makes a unique observation, there is resistance, and then the work snowballs, becomes competitive, and is carried on by others. He is grateful for the chance to contribute, and has no regrets for his devotion to his idea, but only for the burden of insecurity and stress that that devotion placed on his family.

Must it be this way? Unfortunately, there are no signs of change in the scientific establishment or the ways in which research is recognized and funded. If anything, the waters are becoming more muddied, with many researchers complaining that their work is being influenced by drug companies and special-interest groups. The cholesterol lobby is still powerful; when a group of scientists proposed recently that it is not cost-effective, and perhaps not even safe, to test and treat people under thirty-five for high blood cholesterol, the scientists were confronted with a firestorm of criticism from cholesterol-theory proponents.

Perhaps McCully is right, after all, to consider himself lucky. He now has a forum for his ideas and a way to influence public health through information. As he remarked to me more than once, not everyone gets to do what they grew up wanting to do. In his case, he went into medicine in order to apply basic science—especially chemistry, his specialty—to the problems of human disease. At that, he has ultimately—and spectacularly—succeeded.

—Michelle Stacey,
author of "The Fall and Rise of Kilmer McCully,"
New York Times Magazine, August 9, 1997,
and author of *Consumed: Why Americans Love,
Hate, and Fear Food*

1

What Is Homocysteine?

What you believe about heart disease is about to change. Many Americans, including medical scientists, have a one-track mind when it comes to the condition. In the past, fats and cholesterol in the diet were blamed for causing heart disease. But years of medical research have produced no convincing evidence that these components of foods actually cause hardening of the arteries. In fact, scientists have proven that pure cholesterol does not cause arteriosclerosis and that elevation of blood cholesterol is a symptom—not a cause—of heart disease. Discoveries about a substance in our bodies, homocysteine, are revolutionizing our understanding of the cause of the nation's number one killer. We have learned that deficiencies of B vitamins in the diet—folic acid, vitamin B6, vitamin B12—trigger heart disease by raising the level of homocysteine in the blood. Now there is a way to prevent heart disease and to achieve a longer, healthier life. All you have to do is improve your diet.

These simple yet revolutionary discoveries and concepts are very different from what we've been told for years. Heart disease has been studied, researched, and discussed, and yet it's still the number one killer in this country. How could all the medical experts be wrong about something this big, this important? Could we experience a revolution in our thinking in this day and age? We understand how Copernicus changed the way we viewed the Earth, not as the center of the universe, but as a planet revolving around the sun. That's how the word "revolution" took on its profound meaning. But that was five hundred years ago, and there was less information available in those days. Certainly today we would know if the experts were off base. Maybe not.

There is a revolution going on. The way we look at disease and aging, especially heart disease, is changing. The previously touted dangers of dietary fats and cholesterol need to be reconsidered, and existing theories need to be revised because of the new discoveries about homocysteine and heart disease.

In the past few decades, deaths from heart disease have actually gone down. Why? The National Institutes of Health can't explain it. Our eating habits have not improved; in fact they've gotten worse. We eat more fat and cholesterol than ever and our blood cholesterol levels are up. The experts can't explain declining deaths from heart disease in terms of medical therapy, or changes in smoking or exercise patterns. Is it possible the cholesterol theory is just plain wrong?

There are more unanswered questions. How do we explain that a large percentage of patients with heart disease have normal cholesterol levels? Or that the French, who love pâté de foie gras and red wine, have a much lower incidence of heart disease than do abstemious Americans? Or that Eskimos of Greenland or the Masai of Africa who eat meat-based diets have almost no heart disease? No one has been able to explain these paradoxes. Until now.

The millions of research dollars spent trying to prove the cholesterol theory have all come up empty-handed. The eighty-five-year reign of the cholesterol theory of heart disease is coming to an end. Our thinking has to change.

In this book I will present a totally new way of looking at the nation's number one killer, heart disease. Homocysteine, an amino acid present in our bodies, has been identified as the cause of heart disease—as well as blood clots, stroke, and gangrene. The homocysteine theory of heart disease has gained attention because it has been proven—sometimes by the very studies that were trying to validate the cholesterol theory. What's more, keeping homocysteine levels in the safe range doesn't require expensive medication or any drugs at all, only adequate amounts of certain vitamins—B6, B12, and folic acid—from fresh whole foods.

I'll explain how homocysteine causes heart disease and the role of B vitamins in keeping homocysteine levels in check. I'll show how the processing and refining of foods destroys these vitamins. I'll document that the U.S. population overall is deficient in B vitamins as a result. I'll show that the reason the cholesterol in LDL is dangerous is that it carries homocysteine to arteries. It's a matter of life and death that we control the level of homocysteine in our blood.

This book will also look at the relationship between homocysteine and the risk factors we know about, such as smoking, heredity, lack of exercise, hormones, and aging. But this book is not just about heart disease. Homocysteine is intimately involved in the aging process and certain other diseases, including Alzheimer's, arthritis, and cancer.

Since I began my research thirty years ago, hundreds of research papers have been published that validate my homocysteine theory. If you're interested in knowing about the revolution that's been taking place, you'll be fascinated to learn about homocysteine and the role it plays in the body. You don't have to worry that it's speculation, or some untested idea. It's proven.

The best part is that you can do something about your homocysteine level. Easily. I will show you how to eat a diet that is rich in B vitamins, phytochemicals, minerals, and other nutrients that prevent homocysteine buildup. As a result, you'll completely avoid heart disease and all the related conditions. It's that simple. You can find out your current homocysteine level by asking your doctor to do a blood test. If your homocysteine is low (6–8 micromoles per liter), you are at low risk of developing heart disease. If your homocysteine level is elevated (anything over 12 micromoles per liter), you can reduce it to a safe level by eating the nutritious Heart Revolution diet.

The Case for the Heart Revolution Diet

Before I explain the creation of the homocysteine theory of heart disease, the following case studies will illustrate how two individuals have improved their health by following the Heart Revolution diet. These experiments show how eating an optimal diet and taking simple B vitamin supplements (folic acid and vitamin B6) were successful in causing weight loss, lowering blood pressure, lowering blood homocysteine levels, reducing heart disease symptoms, and improving general health.

Case Study #1

In 1983, J.E., a moderately obese, hard-driving, cigarette-smoking, middle-management executive, age forty-two, suffered an episode of intense chest pain. During hospitalization, he was found to have had a typical myocardial infarction (heart attack) caused by thrombosis of the coronary artery (blockage of an artery to the heart by blood clots). His blood cholesterol was 195 milligrams per deciliter—a figure in the desirable range. His blood pressure was normal. Following an uneventful recovery from his heart attack, he gave up smoking and tried to lose weight by adopting a low-fat, low-cholesterol diet.

No further symptoms were noticed until 1994, when at age fifty-three, he started gaining weight and developed acute chest pain felt on exertion. An angiogram X-ray of his coronary arteries showed partial blockage and narrowing of his left coronary artery. He was treated successfully with balloon angioplasty, a procedure to open the artery, and his symptoms of chest discomfort were relieved. His blood cholesterol was now 230 milligrams per deciliter, slightly high, so his doctor prescribed pravastatin, which lowered his cholesterol to 185. The blood homocysteine level was also measured and found to be 21 micromoles per liter, which is very high. Because of stomach and liver prob-

lems, he was taken off pravastatin. He was still getting fatter (his weight was now at 242 pounds). Because his blood sugar levels were now slightly elevated he was given chlorpropamide, a drug for treating adult-onset diabetes. Clearly, J.E. was very ill and was not improving with standard therapies.

When J.E. learned of the Heart Revolution diet and the homocysteine theory of arteriosclerosis, he began taking 1 milligram of folic acid and 25 milligrams of vitamin B6 per day. He cut way back on refined carbohydrates (soft drinks, white bread, pasta, white rice, and desserts) and started eating more vegetables, fruits, fish, and lean meats. After one year on this program, he had lost nine pounds, and his diabetes improved. His homocysteine level fell to 12. The results of a stress test done at this time were normal, indicating good circulation. The best news was that he was able to stop taking all medications. At age fifty-seven, J.E. is markedly better and is continuing the Heart Revolution diet and supplemental vitamins.

Case Study #2

Beginning in 1991, R.S., a sixty-two-year-old, slightly obese, nonsmoking executive in excellent health started gaining weight. At a routine checkup, he tipped in at 226 pounds, and his blood pressure was higher than in the preceding five years. His blood homocysteine level was 10.6. Because of his weight gain, he found it harder to exercise.

R.S. began the Heart Revolution diet and started taking one or two multivitamin tablets per day. He also eliminated white flour, pasta, bagels, crackers, soft drinks, beer, and desserts from his diet, replacing these foods with ten servings of fruits and vegetables per day. He began eating fish twice per week and ate four servings per week of lean poultry and meat. Carbohydrates from potatoes, brown rice, oatmeal, and whole wheat were limited to three or four servings per week.

After two years on this program R.S. had lost twenty-three pounds and his blood pressure decreased to a normal range. Most significantly, his homocysteine level dropped to 7.3. As a result of following the Heart Revolution program over a period of two years, R.S. is now able to exercise regularly, and he just feels better.

How It All Began: The Creation of the Homocysteine Theory of Heart Disease

It's not enough for a scientist to be observant. He must be able to understand the significance of a discovery. Louis Pasteur's famous dictum, "In scientific research, chance favors the prepared mind," emphasizes this ability. In the case of the homocysteine theory of heart disease, I was ready. I had the experience and education in biochemistry, genetics, and pathology that enabled me to understand the significance of something I observed in 1968.

At a human genetics conference that year, I learned about a newly discovered disease, homocystinuria, in which the amino acid homocysteine, normally present in trace amounts in our blood, is found in large amounts in the urine of mentally retarded children. The mother of a nine-year-old girl with the disease told the pediatricians that the girl's uncle had died in childhood of a similar disease in the 1930s. The uncle was an eight-year-old mentally retarded boy who had died of a stroke in childhood. How could an eight-year-old have died the way old people do? His case was so interesting that it was published in the *New England Journal of Medicine* in 1933. The pathologist found that the arteries to the patient's brain were narrowed and blocked by a blood clot, causing the stroke that killed him. The pathologist commented that the arteries looked like arteriosclerosis (hardening of the arteries) usually found in the elderly.

Coincidentally, the case from 1933 had been published from the department where I was currently working at the Massachusetts General Hospital, so I decided to restudy it. The archives contained the original autopsy report, microscopic slides, and small fragments of his organs preserved in paraffin. My study confirmed that the boy had arteriosclerosis in many arteries throughout his body—similar to the arteriosclerosis that I had seen in elderly patients. But it was amazing that there was no cholesterol or fat deposited in the arteriosclerotic plaques in this child. This boy had the disease homocystinuria, and I reasoned that the amino acid homocysteine could have produced the arteriosclerosis and stroke by damaging artery walls. I interpreted this fascinating case to indicate that rapidly progressive severe damage to arteries can occur *before* fats and cholesterol are deposited in arteriosclerotic plaques.

Several months later, I learned of another recent case of homocystinuria in a two-month-old baby boy. The child hadn't been growing properly and had died of severe pneumonia. This baby also had homocysteine in his urine and was found to have a previously unknown form of the disease caused by a problem with the function of vitamin B12 and folic acid in his body. An autopsy had been performed when the child died, and the completed report was filed in our departmental archives. Because the case from 1933 was caused by a different problem with another vitamin, vitamin B6, the condition of the arteries in this recent case was crucial. If the arteries were found to be free of arteriosclerosis, the case would show that blood homocysteine could be highly elevated without damaging the arteries. If the arteries were found to contain arteriosclerotic plaques, it would prove that homocysteine causes damage to arteries regardless of which condition caused elevation of blood homocysteine.

When I read the second crucial case, I found no mention of the arteries in the description of the findings. There were two possibilities. Either the pathologist who completed the case had not found the changes in the arteries, or the arteries were in fact normal. But when I made a detailed study of this second case, I discovered that this child also had rapidly progressive arteriosclerosis, just as I had predicted!

I barely slept for two weeks. I became very excited because my analysis of these two cases of homocystinuria proved that the amino acid *homocysteine was causing arteriosclerosis by directly damaging the cells and tissues of the arteries*. Since one case resulted from a lack of vitamin B6 and the other from a deficiency in B12 and folic acid, I could pinpoint the one constant—a high level of homocysteine in the blood—as the factor responsible for the arteriosclerosis. If this amino acid produced arteriosclerosis in these patients, then why couldn't homocysteine cause the disease in the rest of the population?

I immediately thought of other well-known experiments that were relevant. In 1949 the California pathologist James Rinehart did some experiments on monkeys showing that when vitamin B6 is limited in the diet, the result is arteriosclerosis. Rinehart had linked a B6 deficiency with the disease, but he couldn't explain exactly how they were related. Suddenly I realized that the missing link was homocysteine. The B6 deficiency raised homocysteine levels, and that's how arteriosclerosis was caused in Rinehart's monkeys. In other studies from Canada, involving experiments with rats, vitamins B12 and folic acid prevented arteriosclerosis. Again the missing link was homocysteine. I knew that B12 and folic acid controlled homocysteine, and if there were enough of these vitamins, homocysteine would be kept low, therefore preventing the disease.

This was a powerful discovery. It showed that vitamins could help prevent heart disease by controlling homocysteine—not only in rare cases of homocystinuria and in experimental animals, but also in the rest of us. If you look at the American diet, it's easy to see that we don't get enough B vitamins. We eat processed foods that don't provide the vitamins our bodies need. As a result, homocysteine goes up, arteries are damaged, and heart disease takes over.

The biochemist Albert Szent-Gyorgi described scientific discovery as a process that begins with analysis of the same facts that other scientists examine, but concludes with a new concept based on fresh observation. Certainly, this was a new way of looking at an old problem.

The Heart of the Theory

In 1969 I first proposed the homocysteine theory of heart disease. When there is too much homocysteine in the blood, arteries are damaged and plaques form. The result is arteriosclerosis and heart disease. This happens when we don't get enough of certain vitamins—namely B6, B12, and folic acid. These B vitamins are missing in our diets because processing and refining foods (think white flour, sugar, and canning) destroys these sensitive vitamins.

When I first started my research, homocysteine was an obscure minor amino acid known only to biochemists for its function in protein metabolism. Before the disease homocystinuria was discovered in 1962, medical scientists had no clue that homocysteine could be a key player in the most important disease in the population—arteriosclerosis.

Of course, besides diet there are many other factors that can increase homocysteine in our blood: genetic background, certain drugs, aging, hormonal changes such as menopause, smoking, how little we exercise, diabetes, and high blood pressure. We can't control all these things. But we can do something about our diet, and our diet is the one sure way to keep homocysteine levels low.

How do you eat? Is your diet mostly meat and potatoes? Is it low-fat and high-carbohydrate? Are you a vegetarian? A vegan? Do you follow a high-protein plan? How you eat affects how your body prevents disease.

Often it's the balance of what you eat that needs adjustment. For example, an amino acid called methionine is one of the essential building blocks of all proteins in foods. It is especially abundant in meats and dairy products. In the body, methionine is normally converted to homocysteine. We need some methionine, but an excessive amount will create too much homocysteine, damaging the arteries. The good news is that homocysteine can also be converted back to methionine or excreted from the body by the three important B vitamins—folic acid, B6, and B12. So if meat-eaters eat enough fruits and vegetables containing the proper B vitamins, homocysteine will not build up in the blood. But most meat-eaters usually don't consume enough fruits and vegetables (think of the typical fast-food American diet), and that's why they are more susceptible to disease.

Vegetarians are generally protected from arteriosclerosis. Vegetable proteins derived from grains, beans, peas, and other vegetables contain less methionine than protein derived from meat, fish, and dairy products, so less homocysteine is produced in the body. Plus a vegetarian diet usually contains large amounts of B vitamins, so homocysteine levels are also kept low by the vitamins. But you'll see later in the book that vegetarianism isn't necessarily the ideal diet.

The message of the Heart Revolution is simple and clear. Heart disease is caused by modern processed food, and the way to prevent the disease is to improve the quality of your diet. The Heart Revolution diet, outlined in Chapter Four, will show you how to eat foods that prevent heart disease and all the other conditions related to it. When you eat processed, preserved, and refined foods, deficiencies of B vitamins lead to a buildup of homocysteine and heart disease. If you simply consume enough B6, B12, and folic acid from fresh whole foods, your homocysteine level will be kept low and you can avoid heart disease altogether. In a sense, heart disease is a modern disease because it's manmade. If we ate what our bodies needed, heart disease would be as rare as it is in unindustrialized parts of the world. That would be a revolution.

The Cholesterol Myth

Why haven't more people heard of homocysteine? It has been hidden by the very big shadow of the cholesterol theory. The idea that cholesterol causes arteriosclerosis has been touted, researched, and publicized for so many years that, until recently, only few people questioned it. The truth is that *the cholesterol theory has never been proven.* The studies that set out to show a connection between dietary cholesterol and heart disease have failed.

For all of you who are eating a low-cholesterol diet prescribed by your doctor, or for those who are on cholesterol-lowering drugs, this may come as a surprise. But no study anywhere has ever proven that lowering the amount of cholesterol in the diet reduces the risk of heart disease. And lowering blood cholesterol through drugs won't prevent arteries from hardening if homocysteine is high. So how did this myth start?

The cholesterol theory was developed in the beginning of this century when scientists studying the plaques in arteries found crystals of cholesterol and deposits of fats from lipoproteins (combinations of fat and protein molecules in the blood). They reasoned that the cholesterol and fat in the food we eat must produce the cholesterol and fat in the plaques.

Studies seemed to back this up. For example, when rabbits, a normally vegetarian animal, are fed meat, eggs, and milk—foods high in cholesterol—they develop arteriosclerosis similar to that seen in humans. These experiments were first done in 1908 to 1913 by Russian scientists. In 1916 the Dutch physician DeLangen discovered that Indonesian stewards working on board Dutch ships developed arteriosclerosis after eating the rich Dutch diet, which contains butter, milk, eggs, and meat. Arteriosclerosis was almost unknown among Indonesians eating their traditional diet of rice, seafood, and vegetables. Many subsequent studies have confirmed that high levels of cholesterol in the blood are associated with an increased risk of arteriosclerosis.

The key word is "associated." As I'll explain, the cholesterol does not *cause* the arteriosclerosis. These early studies don't explain *how* the Western diet creates heart disease. But the homocysteine theory does explain it. Our bodies are depleted of B vitamins because of all the processed foods we eat. In the case of the Indonesian stewards, there were no vegetables on board, so they didn't get enough B vitamins. A vitamin B deficiency leads to high blood homocysteine levels, damage to the arteries, and arteriosclerosis. Cholesterol and fats are then deposited in the arteries already damaged by homocysteine. Subsequent experiments on animals with homocysteine-damaged arteries show that when butter is added to the diet of these animals, plaques containing fats and cholesterol form in the arteries. This proves that cholesterol buildup is a *symptom*, not a cause of heart disease.

Because of these early observations, scientists decided to study diets around the world for clues about heart disease. One obvious example that seemed to back up the cholesterol theory was the comparison of northern European with southern European diets. The northern diets, heavy in fats and cholesterol from butter, cream, eggs, and meat, seemed to produce high rates of arteriosclerosis and heart disease. People eating southern or "Mediterranean" diets of vegetables, fruits, and unsaturated plant oils such as olive oil, had far lower rates of heart disease. These studies suggested that the fat and cholesterol in the northern diets were somehow to blame for this difference in disease risk.

A study in 1997 showed that blood homocysteine levels are higher in countries from northern Europe, where death from heart disease is common, than in southern Europe or Japan, where heart disease is uncommon. So all along, it was the homocysteine causing the damage, while the cholesterol was getting the blame.

Scientists leaped to conclusions about the role of cholesterol in heart disease because they were anxious to find some cause for this major health problem. However, many important exceptions were found to these initial conclusions about the presumed importance of cholesterol and fats in causing heart disease. Certain primitive populations, such as the Eskimos of Greenland or the Masai of Africa, consumed large amounts of cholesterol and saturated fats in their traditional diet and yet had almost no heart disease. Epidemiologists showed that consumption of refined sugar, meat, and dairy foods, especially the protein in milk, seemed to increase the risk of heart disease. The so-called French paradox points to the fact that the traditional French diet contains high levels of cholesterol and fats and yet is associated with a very low risk of heart disease. These exceptions indicate that unrecognized factors could protect against heart disease regardless of how much cholesterol and fat one eats.

The homocysteine approach to heart disease provides an explanation of these important exceptions. The primitive populations are protected against heart disease because they consume no processed foods that would deplete their bodies of vitamin B6 and folic acid. Blood homocysteine levels are kept low by the rich supply of these B vitamins in their diet, preventing damage to their arteries. Similarly, the traditional French diet, with its abundant fresh vegetables and fruits, liver and organ meats, red wine, and limited processed foods, supplies abundant B vitamins to keep blood homocysteine levels low, regardless of the amount of fat and cholesterol in their diet.

So what about the LDL and the HDL? The risk of heart disease has been tied to a high level of low-density lipoprotein (LDL), the so-called bad cholesterol, and to a decrease in high-density lipoprotein (HDL), the so-called good cholesterol in the blood. But until now scientists haven't been able to explain why. Homocysteine plays an intimate role here, too. *Homocysteine is carried in the LDL.* So it's a good idea to lower LDL, but only because it's the vehicle for homocysteine. Some factors like exercise *increase* the HDL level and *decrease* the homocysteine level in blood, protecting against heart disease.

Let's look at it another way. The Japanese have a low risk of heart disease. When the Japanese moved in large numbers to Hawaii and California, they started eating the American, or "Western" diet, rich in meat, dairy, and processed foods. This led to a dramatic increase in deaths from heart disease. Again, scientists studying these situations jumped to the wrong conclusions, blaming cholesterol when homocysteine was the real culprit.

By looking only at an increase in cholesterol levels, scientists went on to speculate that to lower your risk of heart disease, you need only to lower your cholesterol level. But this assumption has never been proven. The crucial point is that you must lower your LDL, which is very difficult to do through diet as most of it is produced in our bodies. A high

LDL is correctly associated with a higher risk of heart disease because it delivers the damaging homocysteine to the artery walls. So it's good to have a low LDL, so that less homocysteine reaches your arteries.

Americans have become fixated on cholesterol. By now most people can tell you their cholesterol level. You may know yours. Many of us have tried to lower our cholesterol by eating less fat and cutting out "high cholesterol" foods like meat and eggs. But this approach isn't working. Heart disease is still the number one cause of death in the United States.

Many experts realize this. For years the medical establishment has been telling us to lower dietary cholesterol and fats to less than 30 percent of calories. However, all the attempts to prove a connection between the cholesterol we eat and the risk of heart disease have failed. Many studies like the Framingham Heart Study, a half century–old medical study of participants followed from youth to old age, have consistently failed to relate the intake of dietary cholesterol to blood cholesterol levels. Unfortunately you never read about that in the paper because too much is invested in the cholesterol theory. Scientists don't want to admit they're wrong after all the time and money spent trying to prove that cholesterol was killing us.

A Numbers Game: Heart Disease on the Decline

Early in this century deaths from coronary heart disease in the United States were very uncommon. In fact, doctors did not discover the medical syndrome of heart attack until 1912. They didn't even completely understand what occurs during a heart attack until the 1930s, when attacks became more common. Then the number of deaths from heart attacks rose rapidly until the 1950s and 1960s, when coronary heart disease became an epidemic. But in about 1968 the deaths from heart disease began to decline, and now, the incidence is less than half of what it was thirty years ago. If the cholesterol theory were true, we would have seen a dramatic decrease in dietary cholesterol and blood cholesterol levels to go along with the decline in heart disease deaths. But dietary cholesterol and blood cholesterol levels have remained relatively constant during the past thirty years. Sure, some of us exercise more and smoke less, and we have more open heart surgery, but these factors account for only a small fraction of this decline.

The major contributing factor is the decline in homocysteine levels as a result of increased B vitamin consumption. Since the 1970s cereals have been fortified with B6 and folic acid. We've been forced to eat more B vitamins, whether we realize it or not. A 1998 study shows that added folic acid in breakfast cereals causes blood homocysteine levels to decrease in people with heart disease. And we've been taking more vitamin supplements. The consumption of vitamin supplements had steadily increased in the past three decades, and more than one-third of Americans now take supplements every day. Overall, Americans have increased B6 and folic acid intake, which has led to lower homocysteine levels and less heart disease.

There is a logic problem with the cholesterol theory as well. Cholesterol is a necessary constituent of all the cells in the body. Cholesterol is actually made in the liver, intestines, and other organs and is then used to make new cells, to produce sex hormones, and to form bile. The more cholesterol we eat in our diet, the *less* cholesterol we make in the body. Conversely, the less cholesterol we eat in the diet, the *more* cholesterol is made in the body. Therefore, if you restrict the amount of cholesterol you eat, your body will simply produce more. And just because you have a normal cholesterol level, it doesn't mean you won't get heart disease. *Most people who get heart disease have normal cholesterol levels in their blood.* Even if your cholesterol goes down, your homocysteine may be high, meaning that you are still at risk.

Many medical experts are aware of the shortcomings of the cholesterol theory. The very studies that set out to prove that cholesterol causes heart disease have failed. The Framingham Study tried to show that eating cholesterol and fat increased blood cholesterol and LDL—unsuccessfully. A number of major preventive trials in the 1960s, 1970s, and 1980s evaluated the effect of cholesterol-lowering drugs, hormones, and vitamins on heart disease risk. These trials uniformly *failed to show decreased risk of heart disease* when blood cholesterol levels were lowered by 5–10 percent. So the effort to lower cholesterol through the diet may make you feel better, as any new health regime will do. But it doesn't mean anything for preventing heart disease.

The use of widely prescribed cholesterol-lowering statin drugs is another tack that has sent Americans in the wrong direction. In the 1990s trials have shown that the new statin drugs do reduce elevated blood cholesterol substantially, even to the normal range. These statin drugs produce some moderate decreases in the risk of heart disease in high-risk groups. The way this works is that by lowering the amount of cholesterol formed in the body, taking these drugs results in lower levels of LDL. Since LDL carries homocysteine, there's less homocysteine damaging the arteries and fewer plaques are formed, decreasing the risk of heart disease.

But these potent drugs have frequent and potentially serious side effects. In fact, they have also been shown to cause cancer in laboratory animals. In Chapter Six, I'll explain why statin drugs may do more harm than good.

The Evil Twins: Cholesterol and Oxy-Cholesterol

The cholesterol theory does have an element of truth. There are two kinds of cholesterol in the food we eat, but only one of them is harmful. In the 1950s medical investigators discovered that cholesterol containing extra oxygen atoms is very damaging to arteries when injected into experimental animals. Pure cholesterol, containing no oxy-cholesterols, does not damage arteries in animals. The cholesterol we get in meat, eggs, and other foods is highly pure until heated or processed, when some of the pure cholesterol converts to oxy-cholesterol. Fried foods, powdered milk, and spray-dried eggs all contain these dangerous oxy-cholesterols.

There is a second source of oxy-cholesterols—within the body. Homocysteine helps to form these damaging substances within the cells of the arteries, leading to plaques. It's not enough to simply avoid foods containing oxy-cholesterols, although you certainly should. You also want a low homocysteine level so that less oxy-cholesterol is formed in the body.

Additionally, excess iron increases homocysteine's ability to form oxy-cholesterol within the arteries. Recent studies from Finland have suggested that increased iron stores within the body may hasten arteriosclerosis and heart disease. For this reason, some scientists believe that premenopausal women are protected against heart disease because they lose blood and therefore iron during monthly menstruation. Iron supplements should not be taken by men or postmenopausal women with normal iron levels.

Proof of the Homocysteine Theory

In the 1990s the results of some very important studies proving the homocysteine theory were discussed in the national media. Unlike the cholesterol hypothesis, the homocysteine theory has been proven by experimental studies with animals, studies of homocysteine levels in patients with heart disease and stroke, and studies of populations that are susceptible to arteriosclerosis. As discussed previously, the arteriosclerosis produced in monkeys fed a diet deficient in vitamin B6 was interpreted as the result of increased blood homocysteine levels. To test this interpretation, homocysteine was injected into rabbits, baboons, and other animals. Just as predicted, these experiments show that homocysteine causes plaques to form in arteries and blood clots within veins and arteries. Plaques are a thickening on the artery wall caused by an overgrowth of muscle cells and deposits of fibrous tissue. What role does homocysteine play? Homocysteine affects this process in several ways. It damages the cells lining the artery walls, stimulating overgrowth of muscle cells. Homocysteine also releases a substance that destroys the elastic tissue of the artery. The final result is a thickened, tough, inelastic artery wall. With time, the plaques develop calcium deposits. The experiments also clearly show that the fats and cholesterol within plaques are a complication, not a cause, of arteriosclerosis. If butter or cholesterol is given to animals that are injected with homocysteine, the plaques in the arteries will contain deposits of fats and cholesterol. However, the fats and cholesterol are not *causing* the damage, they are only being deposited where damage has already occurred. If no fat or cholesterol is added to the diet, the plaques don't contain fat or cholesterol, but the plaques are destructive nonetheless since they narrow the arteries.

Of course, the most powerful proof is in human studies. Some 10–40 percent of patients with vascular disease in clinics and hospitals worldwide has consistently been shown to have high levels of homocysteine. Up to two-thirds of the elderly are deficient in either B6, B12, or folic acid, as shown by the Framingham Heart Study. Patients with deficiencies of folic acid have high levels of homocysteine in their blood all the time. Others with a deficiency of B6 will only have large increases in homocysteine in their blood within a few hours after meals. If a person is deficient in folic acid *and* vitamin B6, blood homocysteine will be elevated both before and after meals. Studies have shown that folic acid keeps blood homocysteine levels low by converting it back into methionine. Vitamin B6 turns homocysteine into other substances that are excreted from the body in the urine.

Here are some examples of the large-scale population studies definitively showing that elevation of blood homocysteine is associated with increased risk of heart attack and heart disease.

- In February 1998 investigators at the Harvard School of Public Health published the results of the Nurses' Health Study, one of the studies that originally set out to prove that cholesterol was causing heart disease. Instead this study has shown that deficiencies of B vitamins are doing the damage. During a fourteen-year period, 80,000 participants answered questionnaires about their food consumption. The study revealed that those nurses with the lowest consumption of folic acid and B6 had the highest death rates from cardiovascular disease and heart attack.

- In April 1998 investigators from England published a study of 21,500 men who were followed for almost nine years. Blood homocysteine levels were higher in men who died of heart disease than in men who did not. The higher the blood homocysteine level, the higher the risk of dying from heart disease.

- The Physicians Health Study, completed in 1992, showed that among the 14,000 participants, those with high homocysteine were three times more likely to have a heart attack during a five-year period than persons with normal levels.

- In the 1996 Nutrition Canada Study of 5,000 people studied for fourteen years, those with the lowest levels of folic acid in the blood were almost twice as likely to die from heart disease as those with the highest levels.

- A study from Norway showed that among 587 patients with proven coronary heart disease, risk of death is directly related to the level of homocysteine in the blood. Cholesterol level, on the other hand, did not predict the risk of death.

- The Hordaland Study of 16,000 residents of Bergen, Norway, showed that homocysteine increases in the presence of other known risk factors for heart disease, including male gender, old age, smoking, high blood pressure, elevated cholesterol level, and lack of exercise.

- A multicountry study in 1997 showed that the death rate from coronary heart disease is directly related to blood homocysteine levels. In northern European countries, where heart disease is frequent, people have higher blood levels of homocysteine than in southern European countries, where heart disease is less frequent.

The study in Hordaland, Norway, is especially interesting because a variety of factors associated with heart disease were related to high blood homocysteine. Known risk factors for heart disease—aging, male gender, menopause, lack of vegetables and fruits or vitamin supplements, lack of exercise, high blood pressure, and smoking—cause homocysteine levels to rise. The studies from Canada and the Nurses Health Study show directly that death from heart disease is related to dietary deficiencies of folic acid and vitamin B6. The Physicians Health Study and the British study show that elevated blood homocysteine increases the risk of dying from heart disease. All these studies are powerful evidence supporting the validity of the homocysteine theory of heart disease.

There are, in fact, many cases of heart disease in which cholesterol levels are quite normal. Usually these patients have high homocysteine that is independent of cholesterol; remember J.E. from the first case study. In 1990 a study at the Providence V.A. Medical Center showed that the patients with the most advanced arteriosclerosis typically had normal cholesterol levels, and two-thirds of all these patients had no hypertension, diabetes, or elevated cholesterol at all. Only about 15 percent of cases with severe arteriosclerosis had high cholesterol. Eating a cholesterol-rich diet doesn't cause heart disease, and measuring blood levels of cholesterol fails to predict heart disease in most of those who have it.

Another significant factor can affect homocysteine levels. About 12 percent of the population worldwide carry a genetic defect affecting the ability to metabolize homocysteine normally. All of us have an enzyme, methylenetetrahydrofolate reductase, that combines with folic acid to lower homocysteine levels. People born with an abnormality of this enzyme need to consume even more folic acid than normal to keep homocysteine levels in check. If folic acid intake is deficient, people with this genetic defect have a greater chance than average of developing arteriosclerosis and heart disease because of elevated homocysteine levels. If you have a strong family history of heart disease, it is worth checking to find out if you have this enzyme abnormality. Specialized biochemical and genetic tests available in commercial laboratories and medical centers can detect this abnormality. I'll talk about how much folic acid you should take in Chapter Five.

An Action Plan: Prevention and Therapy of Heart Disease

Now we know what causes heart disease, and how homocysteine works. We even know what can be done to lower homocysteine levels, which you'll learn throughout this book. And it's not just for prevention. If you already have heart disease, vitamin therapy can lower homocysteine and stop the disease

from progressing. A 1998 clinical study from Canada offers
the first proof that B vitamin therapy can prevent arteriosclerosis from getting worse. Patients with elevated homocysteine
and arteriosclerosis of arteries to the brain were given intensive therapy with folic acid, vitamin B6, and vitamin B12.
The plaques stopped progressing and the homocysteine levels
returned to normal. In a 1996 study of patients with coronary
heart disease, therapy with vitamin B6, folic acid, B12, and
other nutrients slowed the development of the disease.

The amount of these vitamins needed to keep homocysteine in check (3 milligrams of B6 and 400 micrograms of
folic acid) is provided by the Heart Revolution diet. Luckily,
homocysteine levels can be lowered simply and safely by
using B vitamins. And it's never too late to start. We knew B
vitamins were important before these studies, but now we
understand *why* they are so vital.

In 1995 a group of patients being treated for carpal tunnel
syndrome ended up reaping the benefits of the homocysteine
approach. This common painful condition is caused by
overuse of the wrist, hand, and fingers (typists and tennis
players are typical sufferers). In other cases the condition is
related to pregnancy, diabetes, or hormonal disturbances.
Patients were given large doses of B6 to alleviate the symptoms. Most of these patients were helped, but the study also
revealed that these patients had a far lower incidence of heart
disease than would have been expected. In addition, the
study found that many of these patients were originally deficient in vitamin B6 in the blood, which for many had produced symptoms of heart disease as well as carpal tunnel syndrome.

All of these examples point to the key role B vitamins play

in the health of the body. But the purpose here is to make sure you get enough of them in your diet to prevent heart disease. In the next several chapters you'll see how the American diet has failed to provide adequate nutrients. You'll also read about ways to improve your diet so that you can protect yourself.

The American public is ready for a revolutionary way of thinking. Once we change our ideas about what causes heart disease, we can improve our diets, prevent disease, and live the healthier life that is within our grasp.

Glossary of Terms

Arteriosclerosis: Literally, hardening of the wall of the arteries. The muscles cells of the artery multiply, creating a toughened area often containing calcium deposits called a plaque.

Atherosclerosis: Advanced form of arteriosclerosis complicated by deposits of cholesterol, fats, and blood clots within the plaques of the artery walls.

Blood clot: Coagulated blood that forms over a plaque in an artery or within a vein.

Coronary artery: One of two main arteries that supplies blood to the heart muscle so it can function.

Coronary heart disease: Inability of the heart to function normally because of narrowing or blockage of the arteries that supply blood to the heart itself.

Diabetes: Condition resulting from too little insulin (Type I diabetes) or resistance to the effects of insulin (Type II diabetes). Blood sugar remains high as a result. There is an increased risk of arteriosclerosis.

Embolism: Process in which a blood clot breaks off and travels into another part of the body, such as the lungs, brain, or kidney.

Gangrene: Death of the toe or foot caused by a blockage of blood flow when an artery is narrowed by arteriosclerosis.

Gout: Condition in which uric acid is overproduced in the body, resulting in arthritis and kidney failure. Acute gout causes pain in the big toe.

Heart attack: Cessation of heart function when the heart muscle suddenly dies. This happens when a blood clot forms over a plaque, blocking the passageway for blood to reach the heart muscle.

Heart disease: Any abnormality of the heart that decreases the ability of the heart to pump blood. Usually, the result of coronary arteriosclerosis.

Heart failure: Gradual failure of the heart's ability to pump blood. The heart then expands and can no longer run the circulatory system. Fluid then accumulates in the body, eventually leading to death.

Hemorrhagic stroke: Stroke complicated by bleeding into the brain.

Homocysteine: Amino acid found in the body. Normally present in small amounts, it is used in metabolism. Too much homocysteine damages arteries.

Hypertension: Condition of sustained high blood pressure.

Methionine: An amino acid, or building block of protein, that is needed for normal growth. Methionine is turned into homocysteine in the body.

Plaque: Localized area of thickened tough artery wall that causes narrowing of artery and a reduced flow of blood.

Stroke: Sometimes referred to as a brain attack, the formation of a blood clot over a plaque that blocks the passage of blood to the brain, causing death of part of the brain.

Thrombosis: Formation of blood clots within arteries or veins.

2

Why the Low-Cholesterol, Low-Fat Diet Isn't Working

The Carbohydrate Myth

What the average American eats in one day—cereal for breakfast, a doughnut and coffee midmorning, cold cuts on white bread for lunch, potato chips and soda as a snack, and a burger and fries for dinner, followed by a double-swirl soft-serve ice cream cone—is a stomach-turning proposition. Even health-conscious eaters who use skim milk on their cereal, replace the doughnut with a plain bagel, eat nonfat pretzels instead of chips, have pasta for dinner, and eat fat-free frozen yogurt with cookies for dessert, all in the name of good nutrition, are fooling themselves. By eating low-fat foods filled with sugar and white flour and snacking on highly processed, high-calorie foods depleted of all nutrients, Americans are depriving themselves of vitamins, minerals, fiber, essential oils, and phytochemicals that are needed to prevent disease.

We've been bombarded by nutritional information, and sorting it out seems to require some kind of advanced degree. We don't know what to eat anymore. As a result, our eating habits have contributed to an epidemic of obesity, hypertension, diabetes, and heart disease. We're killing ourselves with our food.

The more information that's out there, the more confused we become. Should we or shouldn't we take supplements? Is pasta really bad for you? Should we follow the Food Pyramid or a high-protein diet? How much fat and cholesterol is safe? What's the difference between the two anyway?

Even within the medical community, experts can't agree on which foods cause or prevent disease, despite decades of nutritional surveys and population studies. And there are a lot of myths out there—especially about fats and cholesterol.

The very organizations that are supposed to help us understand how our food relates to our health have presented misleading, often contradictory information. The official dietary recommendations made by the U.S. Department of Agriculture; the National Heart, Lung, and Blood Institute; and the American Heart Association lead us to believe that eating a "balanced diet" in line with the Food Pyramid will provide all the nutrients we need. This simply is not true.

Part of the problem is the reign of the eighty-five-year-old cholesterol theory on which the low-fat, low-cholesterol diet is based. We've grounded the American diet on a hypothesis that isn't solid. There's a perception that high-fat, high-cholesterol foods are the sources of all nutritional evils. Many food and drug manufacturers, eager to make a profit, fuel this paranoia. The U.S. Department of Agriculture Food Pyramid, as a result of our fear of cholesterol, wildly exaggerates the importance of carbohydrates, which erroneously have become known as health foods.

The truth is that only carbohydrates from whole foods are healthy, but the impression remains that any carbohydrate calorie is better than a fat calorie. By not pointing out the difference between refined carbohydrates and those from whole foods, the Food Pyramid encourages us to eat highly processed flours and sugars that are virtually devoid of vitamins, minerals, fiber, oils, and phytochemicals.

The real problem is that the American food supply, which is predominantly processed and refined, is seriously lacking the vitamins, minerals, essential oils, fiber, and botanical agents that actually prevent disease. But we're lucky. We can avoid eating these foods if we want to. It's all a matter of choice.

Building the Food Pyramid

Americans are used to federal agencies and experts trying to tell us what we should eat. The first food guide, *Foods: Nutritive Value and Cost, Farmers Bulletin No. 23*, was published a century ago by the U.S. Department of Agriculture. The guide talked about protein, fat, carbohydrate, total minerals, and calories in commonly available foods. It recommended variety, balance, and moderation and avoidance of the "evils of overeating." It stated ". . . for the great majority of people in good health, the ordinary food materials—meats, fish, eggs, milk, butter, cheese, sugar, flour, meal, and potatoes and other vegetables—make a fitting diet, and the main question is to use them in the kinds and proportions fitted to the actual needs of the body." They didn't get into what those needs were exactly.

Since then, food guides have tried to specify our bodies' requirements and the best foods to fulfill them. These guides have always come from the U.S. Department of Agriculture, and they've typically listed foods by groups and added a few menus and recipes. Some previous guides are *The Basic Four* from the 1950–70 period, the *Hassle-Free Diet* from 1979, and of course the *Food Guide Pyramid* from 1985 to the present.

When vitamins were discovered and nutritional science developed in the early 1900s, the RDA (Recommended Dietary Allowance) was created. The RDA of a nutrient or vitamin is the optimum amount we should consume each day. The Food and Nutrition Board of the National Research Council of the National Academy of Sciences sets the RDA for each nutrient. The first edition of RDAs was published in 1943, and the eleventh edition came out in 1998.

The Food Pyramid is designed to suggest a diet that is nutritionally balanced and provides the RDAs of all known nutrients. In figuring out the amounts and types of foods that should be recommended, the opinions of nutrition experts, disease epidemiologists, and medical scientists are considered. Although most of us don't follow the guidelines to a T, nutritionists, dietitians, and food manufacturers refer to the pyramid in making their own recommendations. The pyramid's suggestions enter our consciousness and serve as a standard for what is right and wrong in our diets, what is healthy and unhealthy.

There are a couple of problems with using the Food Pyramid as the gold standard. First, the economically powerful food industry often influences the guidelines of the Food Pyramid. The various councils, from beef to egg to soybean, comment on the recommendations when the pyramid is being compiled. They have vested interests in how their food category is portrayed and promoted by the food guidelines. A recommendation of six to eleven servings of grains per day clearly benefits the grain producers, increasing the dollars spent on their products. An example of this was the creation of the "Four Basic Food Groups" in the 1940s, which was heavily influenced by the Dairy and Meat Councils to stress the importance of their products.

Secondly, these guidelines do not offer the best advice for preventing disease. Most medical experts agree that poor eating habits trigger many of our national health threats, such as obesity, diabetes, high blood pressure, and heart disease. Have the food guides and government studies missed part of the puzzle? Maybe there's something fundamentally wrong with the way the experts are viewing nutrition. I think so. The Food Pyramid, and the newest RDAs, do not acknowledge the important role of B vitamins in preventing high homocysteine levels and heart disease—exactly what you need for your heart to be healthy.

Tackling the Food Pyramid

The direct connection between nutrition and disease cannot be ignored. In the late 1970s the federal government started paying attention to this relationship. The Dietary Guidelines Committee, a distinguished panel of nutritional scientists, was created in 1980. Its purpose was to recommend Dietary Guidelines for Americans every five years.

In the press conference that introduced the first report, D. M. Hegsted, M.D., a professor of nutrition at Harvard School of Public Health, stated, "The diet of the American people has become increasingly rich—rich in meat, other sources of saturated fat and cholesterol, and in sugar. The proportion of the total diet contributed by fatty and cholesterol-rich foods and by refined foods has risen. This diet which affluent people generally consume is everywhere associated with a similar disease pattern—high rates of ischemic heart disease, certain forms of cancer, diabetes and obesity."

This statement, and all the guidelines that have come after it, including the Food Pyramid (the graphic representation of the Dietary Guidelines), lead us to believe that fats and cholesterol are causing disease. But as I've stated, homocysteine, not saturated fats and cholesterol, is the underlying cause of heart disease as well as all the other conditions that fats and cholesterol are blamed for.

The creation of the Dietary Guidelines provided an even more frustrating situation for me. The homocysteine theory of heart disease had been discovered, developed, and published by 1975. But Hegsted and other leaders of the nutritional establishment refused to acknowledge the role of B6 and folic acid deficiencies in arteriosclerosis and heart disease. Instead, the Dietary Guidelines adhered to the entrenched belief that cholesterol and saturated fats are the culprits in heart disease. As a result, fats and cholesterol have been demonized as toxic and damaging.

The current recommendations state that fats should constitute 30 percent of our calories. In the Food Pyramid, fats, oils, and sweets are grouped together at the top of the pyramid with the comment "use sparingly." As we will discuss further, I believe fat intake shouldn't exceed 35 percent, but also that fats shouldn't be avoided. You need fats for the body to function properly. There are certain vitamins, namely A, D, E, and K, that are fat-soluble, meaning they are found only in the fats of foods such as meats, eggs, cheese, and nuts.

The demonization of fats has also led to the low-fat diet craze that has swept the United States and enticed us to eat more refined carbohydrates instead of complex carbohydrates from fruit and vegetables. The Food Pyramid treats all carbohydrates equally. The base of the pyramid consists of the bread, cereal, rice, and pasta group, with the advice "eat 6–11 servings." But there are carbohydrates from whole foods, which are preferable, and carbohydrates that are refined, which should be avoided. Complex carbohydrates found in whole foods such as potatoes, oatmeal, brown rice, and bulgur wheat are full of fiber and nutrients and break down slowly in the digestive system, releasing a steady stream of energy. Refined carbohydrates made from white flour, such as bagels, pasta, bread, and crackers, have no fiber and almost no nutrients. Complex carbohydrates from whole foods are a much better choice, but the pyramid suggests that *any* carbohydrate will do. Most people end up eating refined carbohydrates *instead of* more nutritious foods.

In summary, I believe that the Food Pyramid is wrong on two counts: First, it is based on the false premise that cholesterol and saturated fats are the underlying cause of heart disease. Second, it erroneously implies that all carbohydrates—whether refined or from whole foods—are preferable to fats.

The mid-section of the Food Pyramid describing fruits and

vegetables is pretty good in terms of advice, but I would suggest a few modifications. For example, milk, cheese, or yogurt are good sources of calcium and protein, and the recommendation to consume two to three servings per day is valid. However, I have a problem with the suggestion of eating only low-fat or fat-free products, because there is a risk of getting too few fat-soluble vitamins, the nutrients found only in the fat portion of these foods.

Another area I would modify is the recommendation to consume two to three servings of meat, poultry, fish, dry beans, eggs, or nuts a day. This group is a great source of protein, iron, zinc, and B vitamins. However, putting beans and nuts in this group is problematic, because it suggests that plant and animal proteins are interchangeable. The truth is that plant protein, lacking in essential amino acids, is quite different from animal protein, which contains plentiful essential amino acids. Therefore, depending only on plants for protein is not a good idea because the protein is inferior. I would suggest getting two to three servings of protein from meats, fish, poultry, eggs, or cheese, every day.

There are parts of the Food Pyramid I agree with. Eating more vegetables and fruits, which are excellent sources of vitamins, minerals, fiber, and complex carbohydrates, is a good idea. But then the pyramid recommends eating "more grain products (breads, bagels, cereals, pasta, and rice)," as part of the vegetable and fruit group. Americans tend to eat processed foods *instead* of vegetables and fruit. Isn't it easier to grab a slice of pizza than to stir-fry fresh vegetables? As I explained earlier, "grain products" are, in most instances, highly refined, vitamin-depleted carbohydrates that are also devoid of fiber, phytochemicals, minerals, and essential oils.

Carbohydrates are essential, but we have to choose beneficial carbohydrates—fruits, vegetables, and whole grains—not refined carbohydrates like sugar and flour products.

Parts of the Food Pyramid are sensible. For example, I certainly agree that it's a good idea to eat a variety of foods, consume grains, vegetables, and fruits, limit your intake of sugars and salt, and drink alcohol in moderation. But the overemphasis on breads, cereal, rice, and pasta, and the advice to choose a diet low in fat, saturated fat, and cholesterol, seriously detract from the pyramid's usefulness. The Food Pyramid is based on beliefs that are outmoded and old-fashioned. We need to consider the consequences of these recommendations. Recognizing that our unhealthy diet can lead to disease, and realizing that we can use our food choices to prevent disease, are the first steps in making change.

Heading in the Wrong Direction: The Carbohydrate Catastrophe

Obesity is another consequence of the pyramid's push toward carbohydrates. When we eat too many refined carbohydrates, and not enough of the good fats and oils, we're heading for trouble. We're eating too many calories without enough nutrients. But fat is not the demon. One of the Food Pyramid's main rationales for telling us to limit our fat intake is that fats have a higher caloric value per gram than carbohydrates or proteins. (Fats have 9 calories per gram, and carbohydrates and proteins about 4–4.5 calories per gram.) Obviously, fats are a highly concentrated form of calories. But studies of primitive peoples, and current studies, have consistently shown that *a high fat intake does not lead to obesity* if the diet contains unprocessed whole foods.

Another consequence is disease. Certain populations naturally get quite a lot of their calories from fats—Inuits, Masai, Loetschental Swiss—and have no problems with degenerative diseases. On the other hand, when the diet includes a high proportion of calories from refined carbohydrates—as does the American diet—the population develops diabetes, hypertension, tooth decay, obesity, and heart disease.

To understand why refined carbohydrates can be so damaging to our systems—both in terms of storing too much fat and in causing disease—we have to look at what happens in the body when we eat them. Refined carbohydrates—white flour, white rice, starch, sugar—are rapidly converted to glucose, a sugar in the blood that supplies energy to all organs and tissues in the body. When glucose accumulates in the blood, the pancreas is stimulated to produce insulin. This hormone is responsible for transporting glucose—or blood sugar—into cells. When cells need energy and blood sugar is inadequate, another hormone, glucagon, is secreted by the pancreas. It helps raise blood sugar levels by encouraging the metabolism of protein and fat. When glucose enters cells with the help of insulin, the cells use it for energy and production of fats. The fats are then deposited in our fat tissues. If a person exercises very actively, glucose doesn't build up in the blood because the body uses it to supply energy for muscle contraction. If a person is sedentary, the excess glucose in the blood is stored as fat. When there are huge surges of insulin because we are eating so many carbohydrates, our bodies can become resistant to insulin. Short term, this means we crave more and more carbohydrates or sugar. Long term, this condition may ultimately lead to diabetes.

Remember J.E. from Chapter One. He tried to lose weight by consuming a low-fat, high-carbohydrate diet. The result? He gained weight and developed early diabetes because his body became resistant to insulin. The carbohydrate calories he ate were deposited as fat.

Not only does the low-fat, high-carbohydrate diet induce obesity, but it interferes with the normal release of growth hormone from the pituitary gland. Growth hormone is necessary for growth in childhood, but in adults it is needed to repair tissues broken down by regular daily activities. The proteins in muscle and other tissues need this growth hormone so they can be resynthesized. If the tissues don't get enough of the growth hormone, they cannot be remade by the body. This is the definition of degenerative disease.

Dangers of Processed Foods

The way we process and preserve foods has created a nutritional void. To make food last longer, or to make sure it doesn't spoil, certain parts of the food—the parts that would attract bacteria, mold, and insects—are removed. The problem is that these are the very parts that contain the nutrients we need to prevent disease. This will be explained in much greater detail in Chapter Three.

White flour is perhaps the most significant example of nutrient obliteration. When wheat is milled into flour, 80–90 percent of many vitamins, minerals, fiber, phytochemicals, and essential oils, including B6 and folic acid, is lost. The same thing happens when brown rice is polished to make white rice. When sugar is extracted from sugar beets or sugarcane, it no longer contains any vitamins, minerals, fiber, or essential oils whatsoever. Canning of vegetables and fruits means losses of 50–75 percent of vitamin B6 and folic acid— the vitamins we need the most to prevent heart disease.

The B vitamins are very sensitive and are easily destroyed by heat, radiation, chemical oxidation, and many of the other ways we treat our food. So if you're eating a high proportion of these treated foods in your diet, the greater your risk of vitamin B6 and folic acid deficiencies, and therefore the greater your risk of high blood homocysteine levels and heart disease.

Many studies over the years have attempted to link fat and cholesterol in the diet to heart disease. As I explained earlier, it's not the fat or cholesterol causing the problem. But, in truth, a high-fat diet usually contains a lot of processed foods made from white flour, white rice, and sugar, which can lead to a serious deficiency of vitamin B6 and folic acid. High-fat foods are usually also highly processed foods. Think about cake, cookies, hamburgers, pizza, ice cream, chocolate-covered pretzels, frozen meals—staple foods of the American diet. This is the way we eat. And that's why there is a vitamin deficiency that, in turn, makes homocysteine levels rise, creates damage in the arteries, and causes heart disease.

Another form of processing wreaks havoc on our food. As explained in Chapter One, only cholesterol that contains extra oxygen atoms (oxy-cholesterol) is harmful to arteries. Oxy-cholesterols are created when certain foods are processed. Let's take the classic example of eggs. The low-cholesterol advocates have us believing that eggs are evil. We know that egg yolks contain cholesterol, which is used to make the cells and tissues of the developing chick. In fresh eggs the cholesterol is protected from the oxygen of air by the eggshell and antioxidants in the yolk. Eating fresh eggs doesn't damage arteries because the cholesterol is pure. But when egg yolks are spray-dried in the process of making powdered eggs, oxy-cholesterol is formed.

Spray-dried eggs are everywhere. They're used in many packaged foods such as cookies, crackers, and other commercially prepared baked goods because they are easier to handle than fresh eggs. What's worse, the ingredients label just lists them as eggs, so we can't even tell if they're in the foods we're eating. The same goes for powdered milk, which also contains oxy-cholesterols. This type of cholesterol is highly damaging to arteries and has been proven to cause arteriosclerotic plaques.

It's not only prepared baked goods that contain oxy-cholesterols. Fast-food restaurants are a haven for these deadly fats. Typically these places fry a lot of their food. When chicken, for instance, is fried in cooking oil, some of its cholesterol converts to oxy-cholesterol. If the cooking oil is not discarded after each use, oxy-cholesterols begin to build up in the oil, and any food cooked in it—for example french fries—becomes liberally laced with oxy-cholesterol. Do you think most fast-food restaurants change the oil in their fryers after each use? I doubt it. If you must eat in fast-food restaurants, it is best to avoid fried foods altogether.

The cholesterol in the cream of whole milk also becomes contaminated by oxy-cholesterol when milk is spray-dried to make powdered milk. Butter, since it contains cholesterol, is susceptible to formation of oxy-cholesterols. If butter is heated for prolonged periods (twenty-four to forty-eight hours), the oxygen in the surrounding air begins to react with the cholesterol in butter to produce oxy-cholesterol. Ghee, the heated butter used in Indian cooking, is a classic example. In a 1987 study of Indian immigrants living in London, an increased risk of heart disease was observed. This was traced to their consumption of ghee. The oxy-cholesterol of ghee evidently was causing accelerated arteriosclerosis and coronary heart disease at an early age.

The oxy-cholesterol we eat in powdered eggs, fried foods, heated butter, and powdered milk is likely to damage arteries and cause heart disease. On the other hand, if you eat fresh eggs, butter, milk, or foods sautéed in olive oil, your arteries will not be harmed. For all the nonbelievers reading this, I'll say it again: *Oxy-cholesterol is the only kind of cholesterol that can cause artery damage.*

Therefore, if you're on a low-cholesterol diet trying to reduce your risk of heart disease, what matters is that you restrict your oxy-cholesterol intake. But you know what happens on a low-cholesterol diet. Typically people give up ice cream and eat low-fat cookies instead. A low-cholesterol diet is often filled with highly processed, low-fat crackers and low-fat desserts that actually contain *more* damaging oxy-cholesterol and fewer nutrients than a diet containing fat. Essentially, this is a prime example of why the low-fat, low-cholesterol diet doesn't work in reducing heart disease. In fact, it increases your chances of getting the disease.

Good and Bad Fats

There are a lot of different kinds of fat, and while some are harmful, others are less so. For example, saturated fat in the diet has been associated with elevated LDL levels. Because LDL carries homocysteine, I agree that saturated fat should be limited. But this is only one factor in preventing heart disease. Transfats are a far more dangerous form of fat. These are found in hydrogenated oils. Just check the ingredients labels of packaged foods. You'll see that just about all processed snacks, crackers, cookies, salad dressing, whipped topping, candy, even ice cream contains unknown quantities of these "partially hydrogenated oils."

Hydrogenated oils are chemically altered to contain extra hydrogen atoms. This process stabilizes the oils in the foods so they don't react with oxygen. As a result they last longer on the shelf without going rancid. Although hydrogenated oils are listed as ingredients on the label, they are not singled out on the nutrition facts label the way saturated fats are. I believe these hydrogenated oils are the most harmful type of fat and should be clearly pointed out on labels.

Here's what they do to our cells. Transfats damage the cell membranes, disabling them from functioning properly. Large-scale studies have proven that transfats increase the risk of arteriosclerosis. My advice is to start following the Heart Revolution diet by checking all labels for "partially hydrogenated oils" and forget about eating any foods that contain them. They're not so difficult to give up once you know what they're doing to your body.

Another area of confusion concerns saturated and unsaturated fats. A good way to distinguish between the two is to remember that solid fats, like butter or lard, are saturated, meaning that they contain more hydrogen. Saturated fats are found in foods from animals, but they can also be found in some plant foods. You should limit your intake of these. Liquid fats like olive oil, canola oil, and fish oil are unsaturated and are better choices. In studies the intake of unsaturated oils is associated with a lower LDL level and a higher HDL level, which reduces the risk of heart disease. Margarine is the worst of both worlds. It combines saturated fats with transfats and should be eliminated from the diet completely.

We have been scared to eat any kind of fat. But fats indiscriminately have been maligned. Luckily some hard evidence has called into question the entire premise of the low-fat diet. In 1998 the Framingham Heart Study showed that the *higher* the fat intake, the *lower* the risk of stroke. In a second study the same year of 80,000 women enrolled in the Nurses Health Study, the risk of coronary heart disease went up as more transfats and saturated fats were consumed. But the total fat intake was unrelated to the risk of heart disease. So now we know that eating fats doesn't really cause the diseases the way the experts thought they did. Looks like it's time to topple the Food Pyramid.

Moving On

After decades of listening to health officials recommend a low-fat, low-cholesterol diet, we have seen that it just doesn't work. The homocysteine theory shows why it's inadequate and misleading. We now know that not all fats and cholesterol cause arteriosclerosis, stroke, and heart attack—only the transfats and oxy-cholesterols. Instead, we should focus our attention on refined carbohydrates that are depleted in B vitamins—and so lead to an elevation of homocysteine. These refined carbohydrates are also responsible in large measure for the obesity, high blood pressure, and diabetes that set the stage for homocysteine to damage arteries.

Official guidelines such as RDAs and the Food Pyramid should focus on getting Americans to consume enough B vitamins to prevent the elevation of homocysteine. We know that large portions of the population are deficient in B vitamins—the Framingham Heart Study, the Nurses Health Study, and the Health Canada survey have proved it. An adult needs 400 micrograms of folic acid a day and 3 milligrams of vitamin B6 a day to prevent death from heart disease. The RDA for folic acid was increased to 400 in 1998. But the RDA for B6 is currently 1.3 to 1.7 milligrams per day, which I believe is too low. The Food and Nutrition Board should increase the RDA for B6. Quickly.

Additionally, the Food Pyramid should distinguish between complex carbohydrates from whole foods and refined carbohydrates such as white flour, sugar, white rice, and other processed foods. The pyramid should recommend a decrease in refined carbohydrates and an increase in vegetables, fruits, and whole grains instead. In this way, we'll get enough B vitamins to keep homocysteine in check and prevent heart disease.

I'm hoping that more and more people will become aware of the truth about our food supply, so we can stop believing the myths. With a more balanced and nutritious diet, the mid-twentieth century epidemic of heart disease can become a distant memory. If we work on prevention, we won't experience crises that require drastic surgery or drugs. We can reduce heart disease, diabetes, hypertension, and stroke. In effect, we can prevent the diseases that threaten our health, happiness, and longevity.

Improving the Diet

- Avoid drastic low-fat diets. Don't be afraid to use nuts, fish, butter, cream, and whole milk in small to moderate amounts so that you're getting essential oils and fat-soluble vitamins.

- Watch out for hydrogenated oils, margarine, solidified shortening (such as Crisco), or anything containing transfats. Check the ingredients labels of foods and skip anything that says "partially hydrogenated oil," or "partially hydrogenated peanut oil or soybean oil."

- Avoid all powdered eggs and powdered milk by eliminating packaged baked goods (such as store-bought cookies, pastries, vending-machine crackers, and cakes).

- Don't eat any fast foods that are fried in reused oils and avoid butter that has been heated for prolonged periods, such as ghee used in Indian food.

- Check cereal box labels and buy only those made from whole grains and without added sugar (such as Shredded Wheat, Grape Nuts, or Total).

- Rarely eat white bread, white rice, pasta, bagels, pastries, and bakery goods.

- When eating out in a restaurant, skip the rolls and instead order a small salad, raw vegetables, or a shrimp cocktail.

- Eat eggs, as fresh as possible, in moderate quantities. Discard all eggs after one to two weeks, regardless of the expiration date stamped on the carton.

3

Food Processing

Where Have All the Vitamins Gone?
Why We're Deficient

Isn't it amazing that food can last for weeks, months, even years in your kitchen cabinets? Foods are no longer just picked and eaten, they are created. There are now hundreds of varieties of foods that are manufactured and shipped all over the world. They seem to last forever. But what is the nutritional cost of processing and preserving food? The problem is that our food has been robbed of its essence.

Foods are processed and refined so they last longer on the shelf. Processing and preservation prevents microorganisms from spoiling food, keeps oxygen from reacting with it, and prohibits insects and rodents from eating it. Sounds helpful so far. But the problem is that when we refine food, it loses essential components—the vitamins, fiber, minerals, essential oils, and phytochemicals that prevent disease. Much of what we eat is processed, and I believe this type of food is the root of our nutritional deficiencies.

There are a variety of ways to process foods. Food processing includes milling grains into white flour, extracting sugar from sugar beets or sugarcane, and separating oils and fats from milk, grains, and beans. When we can irradiate, sterilize, smoke, or freeze food, we're preserving it, albeit in a lesser form. Try to remember what you've eaten in the past twenty-four hours, perhaps cookies from the supermarket, pasta with canned tomato sauce, or sugar-coated cereal? If it's been processed or preserved, it's a food that has lost a good portion of vitamin B6 and folic acid—the vitamins needed to prevent homocysteine from building up in the blood and causing arteriosclerosis.

You don't need to eat vitamin-depleted foods. Although the supermarket seems to be filled with prepackaged, cellophane-wrapped, and sugar-coated treats, there is a way to avoid all of them without feeling deprived. In fact, you'll be doing yourself a big favor. Just think, you may be adding years to your life.

We're Getting Sick from Our Food: Food Processing and Deficiency Diseases

Deficiency diseases are not just a twentieth-century occurrence. In the past, major shortcomings in the food supply caused disease epidemics such as pellagra, beriberi, scurvy, and rickets. For example, beriberi, a nerve degeneration illness that results in heart failure, is caused by a vitamin B1 deficiency. Beriberi reached epidemic proportions in the early 1900s in Indonesia and India when rice processing began. Rice in its original form has a husk, which is rich in vitamin B1. When rice is processed or polished, the husk is removed, resulting in the vitamin-depleted white rice we're familiar with. When rice processing began, the populations in Indonesia and India suddenly lost the major source of B1 in their diets, resulting in the epidemic of beriberi. The solution? White rice is now fortified with B1.

Another deficiency disease that's been largely eradicated is scurvy, caused by a lack of vitamin C. In the fifteenth and sixteenth centuries sailors and explorers on long sea voyages suffered scurvy because of a lack of fruits or vegetables on board. Adequate vitamin C eliminates the problem. Pellagra is another disease that is caused by a vitamin deficiency—this time it's niacin (B3). In the early 1900s many Southerners subsisted on a white corn hominy that is devoid of B3. The result was pellagra. Now processed corn is fortified with niacin and the disease is practically unheard of.

As you see with all these deficiency diseases, it's completely possible to avoid illness by eating the type of food that provides the necessary vitamins. Heart disease, too, can be prevented through diet.

A high percentage of the population lives with a subtle but chronic deficiency of one or more of the B vitamins, resulting in heart disease and arteriosclerosis. It's entirely possible to correct the situation. As we'll learn here, food processing causes the deficiency.

Let's face it, our contemporary diet is based on highly

processed and refined foods. Think about the quantity of bread, bagels, muffins, potato chips, pretzels, soda, canned vegetables, frozen pizza, TV dinners, fried chicken, bottled salad dressing, french fries, fast food, cookies, ice cream, and candy we eat. Admit it—a lot. These processed foods contain concentrated calories without the fiber, vitamins, oils, minerals, and phytochemicals of the whole foods they started out as—they are what I call empty calories. Typically, we eat these foods and little else. And that means we don't eat the whole foods that actually contain the nutrients we need to fight disease.

You might think that it's necessary to give up junk food because of the extra calories. It's true, obesity is a serious consequence of this contemporary diet. But it's more serious than just vanity. This way of eating is actually killing us. It's a serious health concern in this country, but until now it hasn't been viewed as anything more than the American way.

What Happened to the Hunter-Gatherers?

So how did we get into this predicament? This is not how our distant ancestors ate, certainly. They were the hunter-gatherers. They would capture wild game and then eat it, either fresh or with minimal roasting or broiling over open fires. Wild vegetables, fruits, nuts, seeds, and honey were eaten right after they were picked or gathered, often raw and uncooked. These foods weren't stored for any length of time, so there was no need for preserving or processing. All the fiber, vitamins, minerals, essential oils, and phytochemicals needed by the body were consumed fresh. This is the ideal way to eat. Even today, some isolated primitive populations such as Peruvian Indians and the Abkasians from the Caucasus region still eat this way. They are often free of degenerative diseases and, in some cases, live to be over one hundred years old.

The hunter-gatherer regime started to change during the Agricultural Revolution, 10,000 years ago, when grains were first cultivated. Before then, grains were an insignificant part of the diet. But with cultivation, early farmers could harvest and store grains and could feed them to domesticated animals.

Basically all the elements of modern civilization resulted from this development. Populations no longer had to migrate to follow the food supply. The productivity and efficiency of farming allowed leisure time to develop technical, artistic, political, and other talents.

Eating grains changed the stature of humans, too. Before grains, early humans were comparable to contemporary humans in terms of their height, strength, and development. The grain-eaters were shorter. The Indian Knoll hunters of the Ohio valley in 3000 B.C. were healthier and taller than the Hardin Village farmers living in the same area in the sixteenth century. The genetic background and environment of these two groups were similar except that the hunters consumed a high protein diet from shellfish and game and the farmers consumed a high carbohydrate diet from beans, corn, and squash.

Flour Power: The Industrial Revolution

These early grains were still quite different from the white flour we eat today. White flour was first produced around 500 B.C. in ancient Greece and Rome, where it was extracted from wheat using stone grinding wheels. A sieve was then used to remove the husks, bran, and chaff. The upper classes ate the white bread because it was labor-intensive and expensive to make; poor people had to be content with the rough, crude flour used in dark bread. Little did they know they were eating the healthier food. During the Industrial Revolution, steel roller presses made it easier to make white flour, enabling the entire population to eat this nutrient-depleted food.

So why don't we just eat the dark bread made from freshly ground whole-wheat kernels? It spoils too quickly. When a wheat kernel is ground, it releases essential oils that immediately start to go rancid when exposed to air. During milling, wheat also releases essential vitamins and minerals that attract molds and other microorganisms. Stored milled wheat flour, even at cool temperatures, will be contaminated by insects and eaten by rodents because of all the nutrients it contains. Wheat kernels have to be milled because they are too hard to chew.

White flour doesn't spoil quickly because it has been stripped of all its nutrients. But every time we eat processed white flour, we're sacrificing our health for convenience. Food chemists have shown that whole-wheat flour has lost about 50 percent of the vitamins, minerals, fiber, essential oils, and phytochemicals contained in the wheat kernel. When white flour is produced, it has lost 80–90 percent of its nutrients. What happens to the highly nutritious bran byproduct? It's fed to cattle, pigs, and other animals.

Sugar, found in everything from cereal to peanut butter to yogurt, is another highly processed food that is devoid of nutrients. In 1997 the average American consumed 150 pounds of sugar—that's almost half a pound every day. Pure sugar, or sucrose, is extracted from sugarcane and sugar beets. During the Industrial Revolution, the extraction process was mechanized, and so sugar became relatively cheap and abundant. The result was a great increase in sugar consumption in Europe and America after 1850. While white flour provides a very small amount of nutrients, sucrose contains *none*.

Corn syrup, extracted from whole corn, is another example of a high-calorie, purified sugar that contains no vitamins, minerals, or fiber. Corn syrup is everywhere. Just check the labels of candy, cookies, muffins, ice cream, canned fruits, ketchup, and relish. You'll see that it's used to make a variety of foods taste sweeter.

Again, using sugar sacrifices health for convenience. Sugar has an indefinite shelf life at room temperature, can be used easily in mass production, and is a source of instant energy. So starting in the late 1800s, sugar became a way of supporting growing populations. Today we live on it. We're so used to everything tasting sweet that many people now prefer a highly sugared cookie to a plain piece of fruit. But sugar is a nutritional disaster. The consequences of eating sugar instead of calories with real nutritional value are severe. These are more than just bad habits—the way we eat is causing a disease epidemic.

Going, Going, Gone: How Nutrients Are Lost During Food Processing

If only we could consume food immediately after it was picked. That's when it has the most nutrients. Of course, it's just not practical to plant your own year-round vegetable garden and pick your lunch on the way to work. So we have to take into account the inevitable deterioration of food once it is harvested, slaughtered, gathered, or churned. The point is to minimize this loss by avoiding processes that destroy nutrients even further.

Many things happen to our food from the time it's harvested to the moment we put it in our mouths. Temperature, contact with air, exposure to light, irradiation, and acidity or alkalinity all affect the nutritional value of our foods.

The biggest factor is temperature. As plant and animal foods are heated during cooking, chemical reactions speed up, causing activation of enzymes, breakdown of nutrients, and the growth of microorganisms that contaminate food. If these foods are cooled or frozen, the chemical reactions slow down, preserving nutrients and killing microorganisms. This is why we have refrigerators. When foods are heated to very high temperatures, they are "sterilized," meaning the enzymes are inactivated and microorganisms are destroyed. This is what happens when foods are canned or frozen. The problem is that high temperatures cause major losses of heat-sensitive vitamins. In the case of vitamin B6 and folic acid, that means a 40–70 percent loss.

Exposure to air is also detrimental to food. Oxygen alters the flavor, freshness, palatability, and nutritional value of food. For example, essential polyunsaturated oils are extremely sensitive and quickly become rancid when exposed to air, meaning that their nutritional value (and flavor) is lost, and the freshness of the food is compromised. If you've tasted bad oil or nuts, you know what I'm talking about. But the bitter taste is only one problem. Vitamins in the oil, including A and E, as well as vitamins C, B6, and folic acid, are also inactivated by contact with oxygen.

Vacuum processing, such as cryovacuum packaging of meats, can protect against oxygen, and so does canning. But canning is a compromise, protecting foods against oxygen but destroying vitamins. The food industry needs to figure out how to can fruits and vegetables without destroying the vitamins.

You may have heard about irradiated food. Irradiation is being touted as a processing breakthrough because it kills microorganisms and improves the shelf life of foods that typically need refrigeration, such as milk. But irradiation also renders vitamins inactive. Up to 50–70 percent of vitamins B6 and folic acid are lost when food is irradiated, the same amount lost through canning and sterilization of foods.

Another form of irradiation is exposure to light. If food is exposed to sunlight or artificial light through transparent containers, the light energy causes several vitamins to decompose. In milk, for example, sunlight through clear glass bottles destroys vitamin A, which is why milk is marketed in opaque plastic or cardboard containers. In olive oil, light inactivates vitamins A, E, and polyunsaturated oils, so colored glass containers are used.

Most of the milk we drink is pasteurized. Pasteurization, the heating of milk to a critical temperature for a specified period of time, was introduced in the nineteenth century to destroy microorganisms. Pasteurization results in some loss of vitamin B6, but milk is not a major source of vitamin B6 or folic acid, so pasteurization is not a big concern. B12 is not affected at all by pasteurization. Infants or young children who depend on the small quantity of B6 in milk should be given formula that is fortified with vitamins.

When milk is sterilized for canned milk, B6 is rendered ineffective. One example of this occurred in the 1950s when there were complications from babies drinking formula. The canned milk in the formula no longer contained any B6 because the heat of the canning process had destroyed it. The babies suffered convulsions. Fortification of the processed formula with vitamin B6 completely eliminated the problem.

Bleaching agents used to whiten flour and increase shelf life also cause additional loss of B6 and folic acid. Now that you're used to reading ingredients labels, look for "unbleached flour," which is preferable to bleached flour.

Hitting Home: Effects of Food Processing and Cooking on B6, B12, and Folic Acid

Both processing and cooking compromise the vitamin content of the foods we eat. But some cooking methods are better than others. Remember, the point of the Heart Revolution diet is to maximize our intake of B vitamins.

Processing meat consists of grinding, combining, heating, and boiling the meats from different parts of animals. The result is bologna, liverwurst, salami, hot dogs, and processed cold cuts. Even some turkey breast is processed, with fragments of turkey meat compressed to resemble a turkey breast. Chemical additives preserve the meats to increase their storage life. The danger here is that the sensitive nutrients, such as folic acid and B6, are partially lost during the process.

When cooking fresh meats, further losses of these vitamins occur. Heating causes vitamins to disintegrate, so the longer the cooking time and the higher the temperature, the greater the loss. I'm not advocating a raw food diet; this is not safe or tasty. But some cooking forms are better than others. For example, grilling allows meats to be cooked thoroughly in a minimum of time and temperature. Roasting and broiling are also good methods, as long as you don't overcook the meat. Boiling and braising meats for prolonged periods of time at high temperatures are not the healthiest methods because most of the B6 and folic acid will be lost. Deep fat frying of meat is the worst preparation because not only are the vitamins damaged by heat, but oxy-cholesterols are formed.

Processed vegetables are one of the biggest problems in the American diet. Canned vegetables are the worst offenders because the vegetables are heated to very high temperatures before they're canned, destroying B vitamins. Food manu-facturers actually sterilize the food, meaning that all the microorganisms are killed. The result is that canned food will last indefinitely, but most of the vitamins are lost. Canned vegetables should be eaten only as a last resort. Freezing is another process that enables vegetables to last longer. But again, their vitamin content is somewhat sacrificed along with their freshness. Unlike canning, though, freezing vegetables doesn't require long periods of high heat, so not as many vitamins are destroyed.

Cooking fresh vegetables properly is crucial. Most people tend to overcook them or boil them in large amounts of water. The sensitive B vitamins, along with minerals, are easily destroyed. Some of them are leached into the cooking water. This is why it's best to lightly steam vegetables, or, if boiling them, to reuse the water in vegetable stock or soup. By reusing the stock, you'll consume the vitamins that have been transferred to the cooking water. Deep fat fried vegetables, such as French-fried potatoes, are less desirable because they contain excessive oils, oxy-cholesterols, or white flour in batters.

The following chart shows what various forms of processing do to B6.

Losses of B6 Through Various Processes

Food	Process	Loss of B6
Seafood	Canning	–50 percent
Meats and poultry	Canning	–42 percent
Pork	Made into sausage	–53 percent
Raw meats	Made into bologna	–77 percent
Raw liver	Made into liverwurst	–77 percent
Root vegetables	Canning	–63 percent
Beans and peas	Canning	–77 percent
Green vegetables	Canning	–57 percent
Seafood	Freezing	–17 percent
Beans and peas	Freezing	–56 percent
Green vegetables	Freezing	–37 percent
Fruits and fruit juices	Freezing	–15 percent
Fruits and fruit juices	Canning	–38 percent

Whole-grain foods such as brown rice, multigrain bread, and wild rice are terrific sources of vitamin B6. Since the nutrients are in the bran and husk of a grain stalk, the goal is to consume as much of the whole grain as possible. Whole-wheat flour, therefore, is always a better option than white flour. Brown rice is preferable to white rice, stone-ground yellow cornmeal is preferable to white cornmeal, and steel-cut oats are healthier than rolled oats. Again, read food labels. But it's important to realize that when a manufacturer claims its product is "whole wheat," many times there is a small percentage of whole-wheat flour mixed in with mostly white flour.

The following chart shows the losses of B6 when whole grains are refined.

Loss of B6 from Processing of Grains

Original Food	Process	Loss of B6
Whole wheat	Made into white flour	–82 percent
Whole wheat	Made into cake flour	–86 percent
Brown rice	Made into white rice	–69 percent
Brown rice	Made into precooked rice	–94 percent
Raw corn	Made into white cornmeal	–87 percent
Raw corn	Made into yellow cornmeal	–47 percent

Folic acid suffers a similar fate during processing and refining. The following chart shows what happens to folic acid when grains are milled and vegetables are canned and frozen. You can see that frozen vegetables are the best choice if you can't eat them fresh, because the least amount of folic acid is lost.

Losses of Folic Acid Through Food Processing

Food	Process	Loss of Folic Acid
Raw corn	Made into yellow or white cornmeal	–62 percent
Whole wheat	Made into white flour	–79 percent
Brown rice	Polished into white rice	–20 percent
Fresh asparagus	Canning	–75 percent
Lima beans	Canning	–62 percent
Green beans	Canning	–57 percent
Beets	Canning	–83 percent
Carrots	Canning	–72 percent
Corn	Canning	–73 percent
		(cont.)

Losses of Folic Acid Through Food Processing

Food	Process	Loss of Folic Acid
Mushrooms	Canning	–84 percent
Chickpeas	Canning	–37 percent
Green peas	Canning	–55 percent
Tomatoes	Canning	–54 percent
Spinach	Canning	–35 percent
Fresh vegetables	Freezing	–10 to 15 percent

As in the case with vitamin B6, cooking methods affect how much folic acid stays in the food. When vegetables are boiled, the vitamin leaches into the cooking water, which is why steaming vegetables is always preferable. Excessive heat, exposure to oxygen, and additives and preservatives can all affect the amount of folic acid in food.

Folic acid in foods is in the form of folate. Cooking and digestion transform folate into a form than can be absorbed in the intestinal tract. Folate itself comes in hundreds of forms, all essential to the body. But chemically synthesized folic acid is the one most written about and is used in supplements and fortified foods. This form of folic acid is also the most stable. The folates of foods are more readily destroyed than folic acid by preservatives and bleaching.

Vitamin B12 is harder to kill. Most processes leave it untouched; however, when milk is sterilized for canned evaporated milk, 77 percent of the vitamin is lost. But ultra-pasteurization, where milk is heated to a high temperature for a shorter period of time, results in only a 5 percent loss of B12. The obvious message here is to choose ultra-pasteurized milk when available. As for storage, B12 is very stable in refrigerated foods.

Not many people are deficient in B12 because it is so stable. But as we get older, the body has difficulty absorbing B12 because of stomach inflammation, various infections, and aging in general. A portion of the elderly (10–15 percent) absorb hardly any at all, leading to memory problems and other mental difficulties which will be discussed in Chapter Nine. A severe B12 deficiency is fairly apparent (pernicious anemia, mental disturbances, and paralysis), but suboptimal levels that are less apparent still do cause problems. Since only meat, seafood, and dairy foods contain B12, strict vegetarians need a source of B12 from these foods or from supplements. If you're concerned or are a vegetarian, consult your physician.

The Innocent Bystanders: Effects of Food Processing on Other Nutrients

The Heart Revolution diet focuses on getting as much of the three important B vitamins—B6, B12, and folic acid—as possible to control homocysteine levels. But other nutrients indirectly control how homocysteine is used in the cells and tissues of the body, and many of these are also lost during food processing. This gets to the heart of why it's preferable to obtain nutrients through food instead of supplements. Foods, especially whole foods, contain many nutrients that are essential to the functioning of the body. These nutrients, most of which are not contained in supplements, react with the body and with one another. But it's not just supplements that lack these nutrients, processed foods do as well.

Vitamin C, for example, controls the reactions of oxygen within the cells and tissues of the body. Vitamin C also maintains capillaries, cartilage, bones, and teeth, and helps our

bodies fight infections and heal from them. It's found in citrus fruits and juices, leafy vegetables, potatoes, cabbage, and
cauliflower, among other things. The highest amounts are in
strawberries, kiwi, mango, and papaya.

Vitamin C also helps convert homocysteine to sulfate,
which is then used in essential body functions, such as heal-
ing. So it's important that we get enough C. But vitamin C in
foods is easily destroyed by contact with the oxygen of air.
Processing and packaging methods that protect foods from
air—like cryovac or cellophane—help to preserve vitamin C.

Riboflavin (vitamin B2) is found in many foods, including
liver, kidney, and dried fish. But just in case you don't eat
those on a regular basis, you can also find it in milk, baked
potatoes, meat, sausage, quiche, cheese, oatmeal, and Grape
Nuts cereal. Riboflavin is used to create energy in cells. It also
helps folic acid convert homocysteine back to methionine,
reducing blood levels of homocysteine. Since this is our goal
to prevent heart disease, it's important to get enough B2.
Most food processing doesn't affect B2. During milk pasteurization, for example, riboflavin is well preserved. But when
grains are milled, 50–70 percent of the riboflavin is lost.
That's why it's added back to enriched flour.

Thiamin (vitamin B1) is lost when grains and rice are
processed, and so breads and cereals are fortified with vitamin
B1. It's also in pork, liver, soybeans, and ground beef.
Although thiamin is not destroyed by light or oxygen, it is
very sensitive to alkali and certain preservatives, especially
sulfites and bleach. If you eat fish or meat that's not fresh, the
thiamin is probably gone because an enzyme in these foods
(thiaminase) destroys the vitamin. Thiamin is used to produce energy in muscles and to promote normal function of

the brain, so it's important. As of now, no specific effect on homocysteine is known.

Niacin (vitamin B3) creates energy in cells, helps control appetite and digestion, and helps nerves function properly. Niacin is found in meat, chicken, legumes, grains, milk, eggs, and peanuts in good quantities. Although niacin isn't affected by heat, light, or oxygen, it is lost when grains are milled, when rice is polished, and when corn is treated with alkali. So fortified foods and multivitamins are important sources of niacin. In large doses, niacin lowers LDL and raises HDL of blood. In this way it affects the transport of homocysteine to the arteries. Large doses of niacin are used on some patients who can't tolerate statin drugs or as a less toxic substitute for statin drugs.

One of the most crucial categories of vitamins is the fat-soluble vitamins—A, D, E, and K. These four vitamins help maintain teeth, bones, and skin. They also are important for reproduction and blood clotting; A and E are especially important in keeping homocysteine in check. They're called the "fat vitamins" because they are found only in fats. When fats or oils are separated from foods, like olive oil from olives, soybean oil from soybeans, or cream and butter from whole milk, all of these four vitamins remain in the fats or oils. So if you're on a drastic low-fat diet (10–15 percent), you probably aren't getting enough of these four vitamins. In addition, these vitamins are sensitive to light and oxygen, which is why, as previously mentioned, milk is kept in light-proof cartons, not clear glass. During the milling of grains about 50–60 percent of the fats containing vitamins A, D, E, and K are lost, and when flour is bleached, an even higher percentage of vitamin A is lost.

Vitamin E is an antioxidant that can help protect against

heart disease. Antioxidants prevent oxygen from damaging cells and tissues, as explained further in Chapter Eight. By regulating the way cells use homocysteine, vitamin E also reduces oxy-cholesterol in the plaques that are formed in arteriosclerosis. Vitamin E is also believed to slow down aging, enhance sexual function, improve skin and hair, and relieve hot flashes and other menopause symptoms. It has thousands of functions in the body, so it's important that we not skip it. Vitamin E is found in whole grains, fish, dark leafy vegetables, nuts, and especially vegetable oils like safflower oil. The problem is that grains lose their vitamin E when they're milled, just as they lose the other fat-soluble vitamins. The vitamin is taken out of foods when the fat is extracted, so a low-fat diet just doesn't supply enough vitamin E. Eating a diet that has some butter, fish, nuts, and olive oil can ensure that you get enough of vitamin E and the other three necessary fat-soluble vitamins.

Vitamin Sensitivity to Food Processing

Vitamin	Function in Body	Effect of Processing	Result
A	Energy, night vision, helps keep homocysteine low	Lost if fats are extracted, sensitive to light and oxygen	Night blindness
B1	Muscle and brain function	Lost when milling grains, sensitive to alkali, lost if meat or fish is not fresh	Beriberi
B2	Helps keep homocysteine low	Sensitive to light and alkali	Poor cell function

(cont.)

Vitamin	Function in Body	Effect of Processing	Result
B3	Energy production	Sensitive to alkali	Poor cell function
C	Regulates energy production, protects against infection	Lost when exposed to oxygen	Poor cell function
D	Allows calcium to be absorbed	Sensitive to light, lost when fats are extracted	Rickets, osteo-porosis
E	Prevents formation of oxy-cholesterols	Lost during milling of grains, lost when fats are extracted	Needed to prevent heart disease
K	Produces proteins for blood clotting	None	Bleeding

Wait, There's More: Loss of Minerals and Fiber Through Food Processing

It gets worse. Along with vitamins and essential oils, minerals are depleted during food processing. Our bodies need minerals for everything from brain function to blood clotting. Minerals fall into two categories, bulk and trace. Bulk minerals, such as calcium, phosphorus, magnesium, potassium, and sodium, are present in relatively large amounts in foods. Trace minerals, such as chromium, manganese, iron, cobalt, copper, zinc, selenium, and molybdenum, are found in small amounts in food. When wheat is milled and made into white flour, 60–85 percent of bulk minerals and 40–88 percent of trace minerals are lost. Similarly, in canning vegetables, minerals are lost. The chart below shows what happens when spinach is canned or when whole wheat is turned into white flour.

Loss of Minerals Through Processing

Food	Mineral	Process	Loss
Spinach	Manganese	Canning	–82 percent
Spinach	Cobalt	Canning	–70 percent
Spinach	Zinc	Canning	–40 percent
Whole wheat	Manganese	Milled into white bread	–40 percent
Whole wheat	Chromium	Milled into white bread	–71 percent
Whole wheat	Cobalt	Milled into white bread	–69 percent
Whole wheat	Copper	Milled into white bread	–70 percent
Whole wheat	Zinc	Milled into white bread	–77 percent

You've probably been hearing about fiber for years, how important it is for digestion, regularity, and feeling full. But you may not know that fiber contains hundreds of necessary phyto-chemicals, substances in plants that safeguard them from infec-tion. When we ingest them, these mechanisms can work in our bodies as well. Examples of phytochemicals include ellagic acid (grapes, strawberries, and nuts), chlorogenic acid (blueberries and peaches), polyphenols (green tea and wine), coumarines (nuts and seeds), and flavonoids (citrus fruits). Among their other properties, phytochemicals counteract the effect of homocysteine in our arteries. As a result, arteriosclerotic plaques are prevented from forming. The presence of fiber and phytochemicals in food explains why it's always better to eat the whole food instead of an extract or supplement. Grapes are preferable to canned grape juice for this reason. However, anything that preserves the fiber and phytochemicals of the whole fruit, like red wine made with the skins of grapes, is beneficial.

Food is supposed to provide nutrients so that we're protected from disease, but processing removes a large portion of the proper nutrients. Sure, we can take supplements, as we'll discuss in Chapter Five, but that doesn't solve the problem. Eating real, whole food does. The truth is that healthy foods are more readily available now than ever before. We don't have to hunt and gather like cavemen, but we have to hunt and gather using our intelligence—avoiding processed, refined foods and seeking out the foods that give us the B vitamins and other nutrients we need. The Heart Revolution diet, which will be outlined in the next chapter, shows how to do that.

Cutting Out the Processed Foods

- Sprinkle a tablespoon of wheat germ on breakfast cereal and eat with fruit, whole milk, or light cream without added sugar. Wheat germ contains vitamins, essential oil, and trace minerals.

- Use an electric grain mill to grind wheat, oats, and barley kernels to produce flour for baking.

- Avoid white-flour products such as breads, pastries, bagels, pasta, pancakes, and whole-wheat or multigrain breads that contain white flour.

- Eliminate pastries and desserts containing sugar and flour.

- Always consume fresh vegetables and fruits instead of canned. Eat frozen produce only when fresh is out of season or unavailable.

- Use small amounts of whole milk, light cream, or butter in cooking and on foods rather than skim milk or powdered milk.

- For salad dressing, use extra-virgin olive oil and fresh lemon juice.

- Store milk in cartons, not glass bottles.

- Olive oil, in dark opaque glass, should also be kept cool or in the refrigerator to prevent rancidity and vitamin loss.

4

The Heart Revolution Diet

The simplest part of the homocysteine theory is figuring out what to eat. The only hard part is ignoring what the health establishment has drilled into our heads about the supposed culprits—fats, cholesterol, meat, and dairy products. As we've seen in the previous chapters, the real villains are processed foods, especially refined carbohydrates, that are depleted of the vitamins our bodies need to prevent disease. Since 75 percent of the calories the average American consumes are from these empty foods, we are not eating enough of the foods we should be eating—vitamin-rich fruits, vegetables, whole grains, fresh fish, dairy products, and meats. The key is to cut out the processed, packaged fast foods devoid of nutrients, and focus on eating fresh, whole, unprocessed foods.

The point of the Heart Revolution diet is to consume enough vitamins B6, B12, and folic acid to keep your homocysteine level in the safe range—around 8. If your blood homocysteine level is below 8, homocysteine will not damage your arteries. And so heart disease, as well as stroke, hypertension, diabetes, gangrene, and blood clots are prevented.

What are the adequate amounts of these B vitamins? The optimal daily intake for B6 is 3–3.5 milligrams; right now the average American consumes only 1.1–1.3 milligrams per day. The optimal daily intake of folic acid is 350–400 micrograms per day; our current intake is 200–250 micrograms per day. As for B12, the optimum is 5–15 micrograms per day; we now consume 9 micrograms per day. If you're eating meat and dairy products, you probably are getting enough B12. For most people it's harder to get enough B6 and folic acid, and even a slight deficiency can upset the body's delicate balance, inviting heart disease. But it's almost impossible to tell if you're deficient. This is why it's important to protect against disease by eating the Heart Revolution diet. In the next chapter, we'll look at the current RDAs of these vitamins to see how even they fall short of what is needed to prevent disease.

Getting Fresh: The Importance of Fresh, Whole Foods

Choosing the food you eat is how the Heart Revolution diet starts. Once you're aware of what's nutritionally good for you, it becomes harder and harder to eat what isn't. For example, now we know what food processing does to the vitamins in our food, as described in Chapter Three. Isn't it harder to pick up a can of processed cheese knowing what's in there? But it's possible to eat foods that haven't been subjected to canning, freezing, milling, extracting, or other harsh processing. Just avoid white flour, sugar, canned vegetables, frozen dinners, packaged cookies and cakes, and all the other processed foods. Check ingredients labels, avoid "partially hydrogenated oils" and long lists of chemical names. Instead, eat fresh, whole foods that come from both plants and animals. This is how to get the largest amounts of vitamin B6, folic acid, and vitamin B12. Changing your food choices doesn't happen overnight, and it's not as easy as just going through the kitchen and tossing out the bags of cookies. But if you focus on what these foods are doing to your arteries and cells, you'll get used to it quicker than you think.

Finding foods that are rich in B6 isn't hard. Bananas, beans, lentils, brown rice, fish, liver, poultry, meats, cauliflower, broccoli, and kale are all good sources. Folic acid is abundant in fresh leafy green vegetables, beans, citrus fruits, brown rice, and liver. Vitamin B12 is only in foods that come from animals, especially fish, shellfish, poultry, meats, eggs, milk, cheese, and liver. Unlike vitamin B6 and folic acid, vitamin B12 is quite stable and resistant to food processing. Because we eat so many animal foods, and since the vitamin is not destroyed through food processing, our vitamin B12 intake is usually adequate. Vegans are the exception. They consume no meat or dairy products and can become seriously depleted in vitamin B12 unless they eat some of these foods or take B12 supplements.

We need to pay even more attention to eating enough B vitamins as we get older. As we age, we tend to eat less and get fewer vitamins. Plus our ability to absorb them from foods just naturally declines with age. Currently the elderly (people over age sixty-five) get only 1.3–1.6 milligrams of B6, 174–220 micrograms of folic acid, and 4.5 micrograms of B12—less than half of what I would recommend.

Another thing happens as we age. There's a special protein produced by the stomach, called intrinsic factor, that is needed so that vitamin B12 can be absorbed from the intestine. We begin to produce less intrinsic factor as we get older. We also have less stomach acid, and the stomach may become inflamed as a result of bacterial infection—all of these make it difficult for the body to absorb B12 and folic acid. Many elderly are deficient in vitamin B12, which helps explain why homocysteine levels in the blood rise as we age.

An Optimal Diet for Health

It's important to cut out the processed foods, but it's even more crucial to eat enough of the nonprocessed foods. To keep homocysteine levels in the safe range and prevent heart disease, the best diet includes six to ten servings a day of fresh vegetables and fruits, two to three servings of whole-grain foods or legumes, and two to three servings of fresh fish, poultry, meat, eggs, or other dairy products. A serving consists of two to four ounces of meat, or a half cup of vegetables. Try to eliminate the highly processed and refined foods from your diet completely. Once that happens, you'll see that you are forced to get calories from fresh whole foods that are good sources of B vitamins and other essential nutrients.

How much to eat is a different question. Every body requires a different amount of food. Adult men and women need anywhere from 1,500 to 2,000 calories a day to maintain a normal body weight. This assumes some physical activity that is typical of American adults. With more strenuous physical exertion you need more calories just to maintain your body weight. A large man working at a job requiring continuous heavy lifting, walking, and physical activity may need 3,000 to 4,000 calories a day. A small woman who runs every day could eat 2,000 calories or more. Pregnancy is another exception; a woman requires more nutrients, including protein, vitamins, minerals, and phytochemicals to supply the needs of her developing baby—about 10–15 percent more calories.

Teenagers and young adults require a higher intake of calories as they grow and develop. An active, tall, adolescent boy may require 3,000 or more calories per day during the growth phase. All too often, however, children and adolescents eat too many calories from sugar and white flour, leading to obesity even in childhood. The problem is exacerbated when teenagers don't exercise properly, and instead are glued to their computers or TVs. One out of every five children and adolescents is now considered obese.

Anyone in middle age knows that fewer calories are needed. But that doesn't mean you have to gain weight. Eating the Heart Revolution diet and engaging in moderate physical activity are ways to prevent that middle-age bulge. Once you are in your seventies and eighties, even fewer calories are needed and food consumption may decline to 1,000 to 1,500 calories a day. The elderly also have a harder time absorbing vitamins, and so they can easily become deficient in folic acid, B6, and B12. As shown by the Framingham

Heart Study, low levels of these B vitamins in the elderly lead to elevated levels of homocysteine in the blood and narrowing of arteries by arteriosclerosis.

Where to Get Your Vitamins

B6	Folic Acid	B12
Fish	Green leafy vegetables	Fish
Meat	Citrus fruits	Meat
Poultry	Liver	Liver
Bananas	Whole grains	Cheese
Whole grains	Peas	Milk
Liver	Beans	Clams
Peas	Nuts	Oysters
Beans		Eggs
Nuts		
Broccoli		
Brussels sprouts		
Lentils		
Kale		
Spinach		
Sweet potatoes		
Winter squash		

A Balancing Act: Fat, Carbohydrates, and Protein

The Heart Revolution diet, designed to prevent disease, is a balance of protein, fat, and carbohydrates. It contains quite a bit of protein (20–25 percent of calories) in the form of meat, fish, poultry, eggs, milk, cheese, and beans. About 25–35 percent of the diet's calories should be consumed in the form of fats, mostly coming from the animal foods that we eat. Extra fats such as olive oil, butter, cream, and fish oil can be added in small amounts. Finally, carbohydrates—in fresh vegetables, fruits, and some whole grains—should constitute 40–55 percent of our calories.

You'll notice there are no added calories from carbohydrates in foods made from white flour or sugar. I know that this diet is different from what the Food Pyramid suggests, as discussed in Chapter Two. Here, refined carbohydrates are absent, and carbohydrates in general make up a lower percentage of the Heart Revolution diet.

We have to change how we eat. The typical American diet currently contains only about 15 percent of calories from protein and 65 percent or more of calories from refined and processed fats and carbohydrates. Right now, the fats most Americans eat are not the beneficial kind, but the fast-food-french-fry variety, which are harmful. Once you increase your protein intake and limit refined carbohydrates, the difference in how you feel is amazing. You'll lose excess fat, have more energy, need less sleep, and, the best part, prevent the deadly diseases associated with getting older.

This diet works because the added vegetables and fruits will give you folic acid and vitamin B6, and the added fish, meat, and dairy products will supply vitamin B12. Homocysteine levels are kept low, and so is the risk of arteriosclerosis, cancer, and other degenerative diseases.

In the next section, I'll show you exactly how to cut out the refined carbohydrates and increase the protein. You'll see it's easier than you think.

The Bread Basket Syndrome: Eliminating
Refined, Processed Carbohydrates

Ever notice how many people sit down in a restaurant, devour the bread basket, order pasta as a main course, share angel food cake for dessert, and feel virtuous in their food choices? We've all been there. The problem is that by eating all processed carbohydrates, we leave very little room for any vegetables, meat, or fruits that will provide the nutrients we need. Not only do the foods mentioned above contain a lot of refined carbohydrates and are seriously depleted in vitamin B6 and folic acid, they unfortunately *replace* nutritious foods in most diets.

Eating so many refined carbohydrates also makes us fat. A typical American eats about 1,500 to 2,500 calories a day in the form of white bread, pasta, soda, desserts, pastries, bagels, cakes, cookies, crackers, and candy that are made from white flour and sugar. Exercising to burn off these extra calories helps, but the surest way to prevent excess weight gain is to avoid refined carbohydrates in the first place.

I want to make it clear that I am not recommending a diet that is devoid of carbohydrates. Popular high-protein diets are criticized because they often recommend very limited carbohydrates. That's not what I'm saying at all. The Heart Revolution diet just doesn't have any *refined* carbohydrates. Our bodies need carbohydrates for energy, and there are plenty of unrefined and unprocessed varieties to choose from. Some of my favorites are sweet potatoes; brown rice; fresh vegetables, especially carrots, beets, broccoli, kale, and squash; and fresh fruits, such as cantaloupe, bananas, apples, berries, and pears.

The Kingdoms: Animal Versus Plant Protein

Is meat bad for you? In the past twenty years, proponents of the low-fat, low-cholesterol diet have orchestrated an antimeat and antidairy campaign. Some people have developed a real fear of these foods, wrongly believing they are causing heart disease, among other ills. This fear is just unfounded paranoia. Not only are animal proteins safe, but they are essential for a healthy, balanced diet.

Fish, poultry, meat, eggs, cheese, milk are important sources of high-quality protein and shouldn't be avoided. They contain an optimal balance of the nine essential amino acids that we all need for nutrition and health—histidine, isoleucine, leucine, lysine, threonine, valine, tryptophan, phenylalanine or tyrosine, and methionine.

You may remember from Chapter One that methionine is the only precursor for homocysteine in the body. It's true. An excess of methionine will cause a buildup of homocysteine—*only if it is not balanced by the proper B vitamins*. The problem is avoided when people eat a lot of meat and dairy products and skip refined and processed foods. Look at the primitive hunter-gatherers. They were protected from degenerative diseases because the fresh whole foods of their diet, including vegetables, fruits, meats, fish, and dairy foods, supplied enough folic acid and vitamins B6 and B12 to prevent the methionine in the meat from being converted to homocysteine. They ate the optimal diet. We know from studying these hunter-gatherers that their diet was responsible for their tall height, wonderful teeth, and strong bones and muscles. They didn't die of heart attacks. They didn't get hardened, thickened arteries. They also had the potential for living considerably longer than we do.

Liver and other organ meats, though not appealing to everyone, are the absolute best sources of folic acid, vitamin B6, and vitamin B12 of any foods. Liver in the form of pâté, or even just plain sautéed, helps to explain the French paradox, the low rate of heart disease among the French, who consume plenty of meats, fats, and red wine. (The term French paradox was coined by proponents of the cholesterol theory. The diet was considered a paradox because they couldn't explain the low rate of heart disease despite high cholesterol and fat intake.) We now know that when the French eat their traditional diet, they consume a lot of B vitamins in pâté, meats, eggs, and seafood. They also get the benefits of phytochemicals in red wine, and nutrients from fresh vegetables and fruits. This keeps their blood homocysteine level low and prevents arteriosclerosis.

The idea of fresh food doesn't just apply to vegetables. It's important to choose fresh meat and dairy products too. Highly processed meats (think about bologna) and dairy products (processed cheese) lose most of their vitamins during processing. Canned tuna fish, for example, contains about half as much vitamin B6 as fresh tuna fish, which is an excellent source of B6. Liverwurst contains substantially less B6 than the liver it's derived from. Powdered eggs and powdered milk, which are used in many commercially prepared baked goods, should be avoided altogether because they contain harmful oxy-cholesterols.

So what about vegetarians who get their protein from plants? Plant foods, such as beans, nuts, soybeans, and lentils, can be pretty good sources of protein. But the proteins are of lower quality than animal protein because they don't have the same balance of amino acids. If you're going to get your protein from plants, it's best to combine different types, for example, beans plus corn, tempeh rolled in nuts, or tofu with lentils. You're covering the bases this way and getting more of a balance of the essential amino acids. You don't have to combine them at every meal, but definitely do so during the course of a day. These foods also contain folic acid, vitamin B6, vitamin C, other B vitamins, minerals, fiber, and phytochemicals, and they are important in any diet. Fruits, green leafy vegetables, and root vegetables have lots of vitamins but contain very little protein.

The advantage for vegetarians is that plant proteins supply a lower level of methionine than animal proteins, and so they're at a lower risk of arteriosclerosis and heart disease to begin with. A vegetarian diet also contains more folic acid, vitamin B6, minerals, fiber, and phytochemicals, and so homocysteine is generally kept quite low. Many vegetarians just don't get enough of the essential amino acids since they're found only in meat and dairy products.

The ancient Egyptian culture, for example, was a primarily vegetarian society. They ate mostly processed grains, vegetables, and fruits. Studies of mummies show severe arteriosclerosis, decayed teeth, short stature, osteoporosis, and tuberculosis. Because they ate so many carbohydrates and not much protein, they probably were not getting enough B12, which would have caused high homocysteine and arteriosclerosis.

Whole grains also contain protein. We may think of oatmeal, whole wheat, corn, and brown rice as carbohydrates, but they are also pretty good sources of protein. Before they're processed, whole grains have a lot of folic acid, vitamins B6, A, E, K, D, fiber, phytochemicals, minerals, and essential oils, too. It's the highly refined versions of these whole grains, like white bread, white rice, grits, and instant oatmeal that are seriously depleted in most of these nutrients. For the most part, when we buy foods in the supermarket we get the depleted versions of whole foods. Even if the package says "whole-wheat bread," there is a good chance that it is mixed with white flour and the amount of whole wheat is proportionally small. You can always check the label of whole-wheat or multigrain bread to see if there is any white flour mixed in.

Some breakfast cereals, such as Total, Shredded Wheat, and Grape Nuts are nutritious because they contain whole grains, plus they're fortified with vitamins, including B6 and folic acid. Cereals that contain sugar, honey, brown sugar, or molasses should be avoided because these sweeteners add refined carbohydrates that supply no additional beneficial nutrients. Neither children nor adults should eat these sweetened cereals. It's amazing how many "healthy"-sounding cereals, like Wheat Chex, actually contain sugar.

Getting Over Our Fear of Fat: Good and Bad Fats

As a country we are fat-phobic. But fats, especially those found in animal protein, have been mistreated and misrepresented. The truth is that we need certain fats for proper functioning of the cells and tissues of the body. Essential oils such as polyunsaturated oils help us resist infections and maintain connective tissues. A low-fat diet just doesn't provide enough of these nutrients for the body. And, as I've explained in previous chapters, fat is not causing heart disease. That's the propaganda of the cholesterol camp.

You may find this surprising, but recent epidemiological

studies have shown that eating less fat actually *increases* the risk of stroke and cerebrovascular disease. Low-fat diets increase the risk of arteriosclerosis because of all the refined carbohydrates—depleted of B6 and folic acid—that dieters substitute for fat products. (People end up eating sugar and flour instead of fat.) A diet that has little protein, such as vegan, macrobiotic, or some vegetarian diets, is usually also lacking in fats unless nuts or soy products are consumed. Therefore not enough of the healthy fats are eaten, and problems can arise even if refined carbohydrates are eliminated from this diet.

But not all fats are alike. It is important to differentiate between the fats that contain the nutrients we need and the fats and oils that are just extra calories or, worse, contain harmful chemical configurations. The beneficial fats—omega–3 oils, monounsaturated fats, and some polyunsaturated fats—are found in animal and plant foods. When fats are eaten as part of the foods they're found in, such as the fat in meat or fish, they're not detrimental. But when excess fats are added to our foods in the form of extra lard, butter, or hydrogenated plant oils, we end up getting our calories from fatty foods instead of eating the vitamin-rich foods we truly need. The hydrogenated fats also contain very dangerous transfats. In addition, many overweight people don't need any extra calories, no matter the source.

Even when we are eating fat from meats, some options are better than others. So-called free-range animals, those that are free to roam and eat grasses, hay, and seeds, are better choices than domesticated animals because the fat content of their meat is lower. Domesticated animals—meaning those farm-raised in pens—are fatter because they eat mostly grains and feed that are rich in carbohydrates, which are stored as fat. They also are fed in stalls or lots where they cannot exercise freely.

There's another advantage to eating free-range animals—they contain more omega–3 polyunsaturated fats than domesticated animals. Domesticated animals such as cattle, pigs, and chickens have more omega–6 polyunsaturated fats, which should be eaten in limited quantities. It's important to keep a balance of the omega–6 and omega–3 fats; they should be consumed in a ratio of about three to one, respectively. Some experts say that too high an intake of omega–6 fats without enough omega–3 fats can exacerbate the inflammation associated with various diseases and conditions, including arthritis, colitis, and arteriosclerosis. The omega–3 polyunsaturated fats also help lower homocysteine and therefore protect against heart disease and arteriosclerosis.

The omega–3 oils are needed to make eicosanoids, hormonelike essential fatty acids that control vital functions such as blood pressure, immunity, and inflammation. For example, leukotrienes and prostaglandins, types of eicosanoids made from omega–3 and omega–6 polyunsaturated fats in the body, help regulate blood pressure, immunity, inflammation, blood clotting, and response to infections. Nuts, canola oil, flax oil, flax seeds, and some fish are good sources of omega–3 fats. Sources of omega–6 polyunsaturated fats are meats, oils from corn, safflower, sunflower seeds, cottonseeds, soybeans, peanuts, and sesame seeds. These should be limited, since too much omega–6 can encourage inflammation, high blood pressure, and blood clots.

Fried foods are just about the worst type of fats. Not only do they contain abundant omega–6 fats, but they have often been cooked in rancid fats, which you will recall contain oxy-cholesterols. Sautéing food in olive oil is a better option because of its high content of monounsaturated oil that is resistant to reaction with oxygen. It also has a healthy balance of omega–3 and omega–6 polyunsaturated oils.

Fats found in plant foods are also good choices. Nuts and seeds, such as whole walnuts, flaxseed, soybeans, brazil nuts, almonds, pecans, and macadamia nuts all contain substantial amounts of the good omega–3 polyunsaturated fats as well as vitamins E, C, B6, folic acid, and other nutrients that help prevent arteriosclerosis and heart disease.

Small amounts of olive oil, and even butter, although they are extracted, are good for us because of the monounsaturated fats and polyunsaturated fats they contain. Additionally, we need some of these fats to absorb vitamins A, D, E, and K and polyunsaturated oils from vegetables, nuts, grains, meats, and dairy products. Without these fats in your diet, it's hard for the intestines to absorb nutrients from food. Women who subsist on salad and low-fat carbohydrates like bagels are in danger of developing serious vitamin deficiencies that result in vision problems, an inability to resist infection, and osteoporosis.

The biggest danger from fat comes from eating transfats or partially hydrogenated oils found in everything from ice cream to crackers to candy. Margarine also contains transfats and should be avoided at all costs. The process of hydrogenation that hardens oils and stabilizes them against spoilage creates an abnormal configuration of hydrogen atoms that *is biologically incompatible with the human body*. These fats alter the membranes of cells, rendering them dysfunctional. This in turn increases the risk of arteriosclerosis and heart disease. Always check ingredients labels to see if a food contains transfats. For example, the ingredient label on a jar of Skippy or Jif peanut butter lists "hydrogenated oil," while a natural peanut butter, such as Arrowhead Mills brand, contains only peanuts. Please switch to the natural and avoid the hydrogenated oil. I doubt that you can tell a difference in the taste.

Too much attention has been paid to saturated animal fat when the truth is that the fat itself doesn't cause the real damage. The artificial transfats, which are everywhere in our diet, are the real culprits. If you want to cut out the fat that's really bad for you, avoid all partially hydrogenated oils and transfats. I'm still amazed that the Food Pyramid and other nutrition authorities don't alert consumers to the dangers lurking in these fats.

Speaking of misrepresentation, cholesterol is a perfect example. Cholesterol is not technically a fat, but it's closely associated with fats. Cholesterol is a steroidal alcohol that helps provide structure to the membranes of all animal cells. That's why cholesterol is found only in animal foods. Cholesterol is not something that we want to clear our bodies of; 70 percent of our brain is made of fats and cholesterol. It's also beneficial because pure cholesterol itself is a potent antioxidant that protects cells against injury by oxygen. That's why cholesterol is a normal part of the body's functioning and is made in the liver.

The cholesterol of fresh, well-preserved, and lightly cooked foods is not harmful because it's protected from oxygen. It's only when cholesterol reacts with oxygen during food processing that oxy-cholesterols form—a chemical configuration that is harmful to our bodies. Therefore deep fat frying, powdered eggs, and powdered milk—all of which are staples of processed foods—are harmful because the oxy-cholesterols directly damage arteries. The cholesterol of fresh fish, poultry, meats, eggs, and milk is beneficial because it contains little of the injurious oxy-cholesterols. Just one more little known fact that you will never hear from the cholesterol opponents.

Beneficial and Harmful Fats

Preferable Fats	Undesirable Fats
Omega–3 polyunsaturated oils	Excess omega–6 polyunsaturated oils
Pure cholesterol found in food	Oxy-Cholesterol
Monounsaturated oils	Hydrogenated oils
Butter, olive oil	Margarine
Polyunsaturated oils	Artificial shortening, Crisco
Room-temperature oils	Heated oils, such as frying oil

Sources of B6, Folic Acid, B12

Food	B6 (Milligrams)	Folic Acid (Micrograms)	B12 (Micrograms)
Almonds, 20	0.03	14	0
Apple, 1 medium	0.02	5	0
Asparagus, 8 fresh	0.09	38	0
Asparagus, 8 canned	0.036	10	0
Avocado, half	0.15	18	0
Banana, 1 medium	0.51	20	0
Beans, navy, 3 oz.	0.56	40	0
Beans, green snap, 1/2 cup	0.08	24	0

(cont.)

Sources of B6, Folic Acid, B12

Food	B6 (Milligrams)	Folic Acid (Micrograms)	B12 (Micrograms)
Beans, lima, 3 oz.	0.58	37	0
Beef, lean, 3 oz.	0.52	8	1.7
Beet, 1 medium	0.03	27	0
Bread, whole wheat, 2 slices	0.11	32	0
Bread, white, 2 slices	0.024	21	0
Broccoli, 1 large stalk	0.27	76	0
Brussels sprouts, 10	0.32	17	0
Cabbage, 1 cup	0.22	42	0
Carrot, 1 large	0.15	18	0
Cantaloupe, 1/4	0.10	50	0
Cauliflower, 1 cup	0.32	76	0
Celery, 1/2 cup	0.04	7	0
Cheese, cheddar, 3 oz.	0.05	11	0.6
Cheese, cottage, 3 oz.	0.04	12	1
Cheese, Camembert, 3 oz.	0.09	10	0.5
Cherries, 10 large	0.06	3	0
Chicken, dark meat, 3 oz.	0.39	14	0.5
Chicken, white meat, 3 oz.	0.82	18	0.5
Corn, 1 medium ear	0.16	19	0
Cucumber, 1 medium	0.03	3	0
Egg, 1 whole large	0.06	11	1.5
Egg whites, 3 medium	0.01	1	1.5
Egg yolks, 2 medium	0.16	12	3
Grapes, 12 medium	0.05	2	0
Grapefruit, half	0.07	12	0
Kale, 4 large leaves	0.33	49	0

Sources of B6, Folic Acid, B12

Food	B6 (Milligrams)	Folic Acid (Micrograms)	B12 (Micrograms)
Lamb, lean, 3 oz.	0.33	6	2.5
Lemon, 1 small	0.01	1	0
Lentils, 1/2 cup	0.60	23	0
Lettuce, 4 leaves	0.06	24	0
Liver, beef, 3 oz.	1.00	174	9.6
Milk, cow, 1 cup	0.07	4	0.7
Milk, human, 1 cup	0.02	9	0.7
Molasses, 1 tablespoon	0.06	3	0
Oatmeal, 1/2 cup	0.06	22	0
Onions, 2 medium	0.08	10	0
Orange, 1 medium	0.07	29	0
Oysters, 6 raw	0.05	48	18
Peas, 1/2 cup	0.13	18	0
Peach, 1 medium	0.02	2	0
Pepper, green, 1 large	0.16	2	0
Plum, 1 medium	0.04	2	0
Pork, 3 oz.	0.54	14	3.2
Potato, 1 large	0.30	31	0
Rice, brown, 1 cup	0.83	36	0
Rice, white, 1 cup	0.26	9	0
Salmon, fresh fillet, 3 oz.	0.84	20	19
Spinach, 4 large leaves	0.28	33	0
Squash, acorn, 1/3	0.15	14	0
Squash, summer, 1 large	0.08	11	0
Strawberries, 6 medium	0.04	4	0
Sweet potato, 1 medium	0.22	19	0
Tomato, 2 medium	0.10	6	0
Tuna, fresh fillet, 3 oz.	1.08	7	16
Tuna, canned, 3 oz.	0.51	7	10

(cont.)

Sources of B6, Folic Acid, B12

Food	B6 (Milligrams)	Folic Acid (Micrograms)	B12 (Micrograms)
Wheat flour, whole, 1 oz.	0.10	11	0
Wheat flour, white, 1 oz.	0.02	2	0
Yeast, baker's, 1 cake	0.20	130	0
Estimated daily intake, adult	1.1–1.3	220–250	9
Estimated daily intake, elderly	1.3–1.6	174–220	4.5
Optimal daily intake	**3–3.5**	**350–400**	**5–15**

The vitamin values for each food are determined by microbiological growth assays, taken from the U.S. Department of Agriculture data handbooks and the National Research Council Reports.

Eat to Live: How to Eat the Heart Revolution Diet

After I developed the homocysteine theory, I decided to practice what I preach. So, for the past twenty-five years, my family has adopted this diet, modifying and improving what we eat every year. Within the past year, we have succeeded in cutting out almost all refined carbohydrates. It's not easy, and we're not perfect. But in general, we eat a very beneficial diet for disease prevention. So far, we're all in good health.

In our house, we concentrate on fresh vegetables, meats, dairy products, nuts, whole grains, fish, chicken and turkey, and fruit. We rarely eat bread, crackers, bagels, pasta, cake, cookies, or candy. We never eat fast food or packaged baked goods. (But we always eat birthday cake to celebrate.) Sample menus for a week are at the end of this chapter, and recipes are in the Appendix at the back of the book.

For breakfast, we focus on protein with a little fruit. An off-white egg omelet, with one yolk per four whites, can be made with a little cheese or ham or vegetable; fish, commonly served for breakfast in Europe and the Middle East, is an excellent source of protein as an alternative. Whole-grain crackers or whole-grain bread made from freshly milled flour provide complex carbohydrates. Oatmeal, yogurt, cottage cheese, or Shredded Wheat with light cream or milk are other choices. A small piece of melon or freshly squeezed orange juice, along with green tea or coffee, complete the meal.

For lunch, we have a mixed salad with protein such as grilled chicken, shrimp, or turkey. A salad can be livened up with nuts, cheese, apple, anchovy, or olives. For dressing, we use a high-quality extra-virgin olive oil and lemon juice or balsamic vinegar. Soup, such as lentil soup or chili, is a good source of complex carbohydrate and plant protein.

At dinner, we eat two to three different kinds of steamed, baked, or grilled fresh green or root vegetables such as asparagus, broccoli, squash, Brussels sprouts, kale, beet greens, spinach, beets, carrots, sweet potatoes, parsnips, onions, or turnips. The protein is in the form of grilled, baked, stir-fried, or roasted chicken, beef, fish, pork, lamb, or shellfish.

When we want something for dessert, we usually eat fresh berries, or nuts with a piece of chocolate that is more than 70 percent cocoa. (Usually from France, this type of chocolate can be found in gourmet food stores.) Snacks during the day are important to keep blood sugar stable; good choices are raw vegetables such as fennel or cucumbers, salsa, nuts, cheese, shrimp, fruit, an apple with peanut butter, or yogurt that contains active cultures, but not too much sugar (about 25 grams per container is my limit).

Serving It Up: Food Preparation and Cooking Methods

The best way to eat food is actually in its simplest form. Raw food, like salad and fruit, is a staple of the Heart Revolution diet. A fresh salad made with a variety of greens and lettuce, including romaine, iceberg, red leaf, green leaf, Boston lettuce, arugula, spinach, dandelion greens, basil, radicchio, purslane, or watercress should be eaten every day. Raw vegetables, such as scallions, avocado, cucumber, tomato, and olives can also be added.

The same goes for fruits. Oranges, bananas, pears, apples, grapes, pineapple, apricots, plums, peaches, strawberries, black raspberries (we grow the wild variety in our backyard) and other fruits are best when they're eaten fresh. If an apple is very waxy, you may have to peel it. Canned, frozen, or processed fruits and fruit juices are not the best choices because they inevitably lose sensitive vitamins such as C, B6, and folic acid. You should eat them only when fresh fruit is unavailable. Fresh fruit juice or fresh vegetable juice are excellent choices. These juices can be prepared quickly from fresh produce in a juicer.

Some vegetables can be eaten either raw or lightly cooked. Broccoli, cauliflower, zucchini, peppers, eggplant, and onions can be eaten raw with dip. If you cook them lightly, they're more nutritious because vitamins and fiber are released during steaming or grilling. Also, because we can chew and digest them more easily, they are more easily absorbed.

Thoroughly wash the vegetables but don't peel them unless absolutely necessary because the skin contains lots of vitamins, minerals, fiber, and phytochemicals.

When cooking vegetables at home, use a steamer with a minimum of water or chicken stock, stir-fry with olive oil, or grill them, preserving as much of the juice from vegetables as possible. Cooking vegetables in large amounts of boiling water is not a good idea because vitamins, minerals, and phytochemicals will be leached from the food and into the cooking water. It's much better to use a small amount of water and even to save any excess cooking juice as a vegetable stock in the refrigerator or freezer. The stock can be added to soup or used in cooking other dishes. Vegetables should be steamed for only a few minutes over moderate heat—only cook vegetables until they are soft enough to chew. When vegetables such as broccoli or asparagus become that dull, army-green color, you've gone too far. Try using a teaspoon of extra-virgin olive oil or butter with herbs, onions, or garlic to enhance flavor. Frying vegetables in oil, or even sautéing them in a quarter cup of olive oil, is unnecessary and unhealthy. Lard, which is the fat from animals, should be limited.

Even meat, fish, and poultry should be lightly cooked. The point is to use high enough temperatures to destroy any harmful bacteria on the surface of the food, but keep the nutrients inside from being destroyed. Fish, meats, and vegetables can be grilled over charcoal or in the broiler for just enough time to heat them. Small amounts of wine, olive oil, or butter with garlic, rosemary, parsley or other herbs can be added for taste. You don't need to add extra salt during cooking, or when eating. Although it's controversial, most nutritionists believe that too much dietary salt may contribute to high blood pressure, especially in those people already at risk. Besides, once you've gotten used to eating foods this way, your sense of taste will be heightened and you won't even need salt.

In home baking, use only the highest-quality whole-grain flours, preferably stone-ground or minimally processed. Avoid white flour, cake flour, rice flour, oat flour, or white cornmeal. Consider reducing the amount of sugar to a minimum in baked goods and in preserving jams and jellies. You can buy an electric grain mill for making flour. Whole kernels of wheat, oats, barley, or rice can be bought in health-oriented markets. The freshly ground flour can be substituted in a recipe for bread, pancakes, or pasta, so you don't have to live without these completely. We recently had pasta made from our own whole-grain flour with pesto sauce made from fresh parsley, basil, and garlic. It was delicious. Until you grind flour, keep the fresh kernels in a cool dry place and use only the quantity needed for a recipe. Kernels of whole grains can be kept for months this way, but freshly ground whole flour deteriorates within a week or two.

Watch out for leftovers, too. Try to cook only the amount to be eaten and throw out the rest. Larger amounts of leftover food should be covered and refrigerated right away, or frozen. If you do have leftovers, eat them within a day not only because bacteria will grow in them, but because the vitamins degenerate quickly. Do not allow foods to stand at warm or room temperatures for more than an hour or two because of bacterial growth and possible food poisoning. Remove stuffing from roasted meats, chicken, or turkey; refrigerate right away; and don't keep it for more than a day. This will ensure that you're eating only fresh foods that still contain adequate amounts of vitamins.

Junk Food Junkies: Restaurant Food, Fast Food, and Snacks

You're probably thinking that the Heart Revolution diet requires a considerable amount of time and effort. It does. But I don't think it's even a question whether it's worth it. It is.

What about the fact that so many of us eat meals in restaurants or fast-food chains? Unfortunately, most of the time, you're not going to find the optimal diet for preventing heart disease at your local burger joint. But it is possible to eat right if you choose carefully. Salads, fruits, and vegetables are usually available on most menus, although you may have to ask about a vegetable of the day and order a double serving. In a restaurant, sometimes it's better not to open the menu, but to ask the waiter for a piece of simply grilled fish or meat with fresh vegetables. I promise, you'll feel so much better eating this way that it becomes addictive.

Fast-food restaurants have tried to pay attention to health in recent years, but many of the foods are of substandard quality. French fries and ketchup are poor substitutes for vegetables. The cooking oil used to deep-fry these potatoes is infrequently changed, and in some restaurants the old oil is never discarded but merely mixed with a new supply of cooking oil. If this cooking oil is also used to fry meats, the potatoes may become contaminated with harmful oxy-cholesterols.

When you're in a fast-food restaurant, a salad is always a safe bet. Ever notice how a lot of these places serve mostly white bread, bagels, rolls, crackers, mashed potatoes, and french fries? These foods fill you up without providing any nutrients. Try eating just the grilled hamburger, fish, or chicken and discard the tasteless white bread or roll that comes with it. Fresh coleslaw, if it's made from fresh raw cabbage, onions, and carrots, is a better choice than french fries. Unfortunately, most coleslaw in fast-food restaurants has sugar added to it, so it's best to just skip the side orders and eat the protein.

The desserts are loaded with empty calories. The idea that frozen yogurt is somehow a health food, especially since it's fat-free, is laughable because of the large amount of added sugar, and even hydrogenated oils. A lot of commercial ice creams also contain hydrogenated oils. If you're in a restaurant, ask which brand they serve. High-quality ice creams such as Häagen-Dazs or Ben & Jerry's are better choices because they use only milk, cream, and sugar. But they are highly caloric and contain large amounts of sugar, so the best choice is a piece of fruit.

It's amazing what you'll find once you get in the habit of reading ingredients labels. Nondairy whipped toppings are loaded with hydrogenated oils; Tofutti ice cream sandwiches contain flour and hydrogenated oils in the sandwich cracker; even healthy-sounding foods like certain whole-wheat crackers contain hydrogenated oils. Packaged cakes, pies, waffles, doughnuts, cookies, and candy should be avoided altogether because they are laden with transfats and sugar.

Junk food, such as chips, candy, vending-machine crackers, dessert toppings, and canned cheeses are just about the worst things we can eat. Most of these foods—and I use the word "foods" cautiously—are prepared with too much salt, hydrogenated oils, white flour, and sugar. Any foods of this type on shelves at home should be discarded in the trash, where they belong.

The Heart Revolution Diet Menu Suggestions

Day 1

Breakfast   6 ounces fresh orange juice
              Half grapefruit
              Off-white egg omelet with herbs
              Coffee or tea

Lunch   4 ounces grilled chicken
              Salad of spinach leaves, sliced raw mushrooms,
                 pine nuts dressed with olive oil and lemon
                 juice

Snack   Hard-boiled egg with raw fennel slices

Dinner   6 ounces broiled salmon with lemon juice and
                 parsley
              Green beans
              Steamed kale
              Half baked sweet potato
              Mixed green salad dressed with balsamic vinegar
                 and olive oil
              Roasted nuts

Day 2

Breakfast   6 ounces fresh orange juice
              Half cup Shredded Wheat with banana, light
                 cream, and 1 tablespoon wheat germ
              Coffee or tea

Lunch   4 ounces grilled hamburger
              Sliced tomato and lettuce

Snack   Baby carrots with 1–2 tablespoons peanut butter

Dinner   Roast chicken stuffed with lemon and rosemary
            Swiss chard cooked with extra-virgin olive oil
                and garlic
            Steamed artichoke
            Small baked potato
            Mixed green salad dressed with lemon and olive
                oil
            Mixed strawberries and blueberries

Day 3

Breakfast   Half grapefruit
            Half cup cottage cheese with sugarless jam
            1 slice rye crisp bread (Wasa or RyVita)
            Coffee or tea

Lunch   4 ounces sliced fresh turkey
            Mixed lettuce salad with walnuts and blue cheese
                dressed with olive oil
            Tomato slices

Snack   Cucumber sticks with salsa

Dinner   Chicken stir-fry with fresh snow peas, carrots,
                and red pepper
            Steamed asparagus
            Mixed green salad dressed with lemon and olive oil
            1 ounce dark French chocolate

Day 4

Breakfast   6 ounces fresh orange juice
            3 ounces fish

2 whole-grain rye crackers
Coffee or tea

Lunch   2 ounces cheese melted on dark multigrain bread
             Sliced tomato, cucumber, and lettuce

Snack   Apple
             1 ounce nuts

Dinner   6 ounces broiled fish, spread with 1 teaspoon
                mayonnaise
             Steamed broccoli
             Mushrooms sautéed with butter and parsley
             Coleslaw
             Coffee or lemon yogurt

Day 5

Breakfast   Quarter cantaloupe
             Off-white egg omelet with grated parmesan and
                basil leaves
             Coffee or tea

Lunch   Tuna salad with celery
             Steamed snow peas

Snack   1 ounce almonds roasted in butter and salt

Dinner   Veal stew with carrots, onions, peppers, and peas
             Steamed broccoli rapini
             Mixed green salad dressed with lemon juice and
                olive oil
             Raspberries with 1 tablespoon fresh whipped
                cream

Day 6

Breakfast   6 ounces fresh orange juice
                Half cup cooked Irish oatmeal with banana and
                    light cream
                Green tea

Lunch   Egg salad with 1 hard-boiled yolk and 3 whites
                Raw vegetables

Snack   Apple slices with peanut butter

Dinner   Brown rice and lentil soup
                Steamed carrots with butter and parsley
                Steamed winter squash
                Mixed green salad dressed with mustard, herbs,
                    and vinegar sauce
                Handful of roasted nuts

Day 7

Breakfast   6 ounces fresh orange juice
                Half grapefruit
                Fried jumbo farm-fresh egg with butter, pepper,
                    and salt
                Coffee or tea

Lunch   Caesar salad with shrimp and anchovies

Snack   Yogurt

Dinner   Broiled sirloin tips skewered with red pepper,
                    onions, and zucchini
                Half cup brown rice

Mixed green salad
Half cup ice cream

Snack Suggestions

Low-fat yogurt with live cultures and less than 25 grams
    sugar per serving
Wasa Rye or RyVita crackers with cheese
Apple slices with peanut butter
Raw vegetables with sour cream dip
Baked milk custard with cinnamon
Hard-boiled egg with vegetable slices
Baby carrots with cheese
Cucumber sticks with salsa

Eating the Heart Revolution Diet

- Regardless of your age, eat more fresh vegetables
  and fruits daily to get 400 micrograms of folic acid,
  3 milligrams of B6, and other beneficial nutrients.

- The fresher the vegetable, the better. Just-picked
  vegetables are the healthiest, then farm-stand
  fresh, then supermarket fresh, and the last choice
  is frozen. Avoid canned or irradiated vegetables.

- Steam fresh vegetables with a minimum of water
  and save any leftover cooking water to add to
  vegetable stock (both can be stored in the freezer
  indefinitely).

- Eat steel-cut oatmeal, whole-wheat cereal, brown
  rice, and root vegetables as sources of complex
  carbohydrates. Try to eliminate white flour, white
  rice, and sugar from the diet.

- Snacks between meals help prevent ravenous hunger. Try a few fresh or roasted nuts for a good balance of vitamins, oils, minerals, and fiber. Low-fat yogurt provides calcium as well as B12; a hard-boiled egg is a good combination of protein and carbohydrate.

- Eat one to two servings of fresh fish, meat, or eggs per day.

- A couple of times a month, have liver or pâté de foie gras, which offer very rich sources of vitamin B12, vitamin B6, and folic acid.

- Limit total dietary fat to 30 percent of calories so that you'll get enough vitamin B6, folic acid, and vitamin B12 from the remainder of your diet.

- Eliminate processed and packaged foods that contain powdered eggs, powdered milk, and partially hydrogenated oils. This will reduce your intake of oxy-cholesterol and transfats.

5

Food Fortification and Supplements

The words "enriched" or "fortified" are on the packaging of a variety of foods from cereal to bread to milk. Most people don't realize that extra nutrients have been added to a lot of what we eat. Of course, much of this wouldn't be necessary if we didn't take everything *out* of food during refining and processing. Food fortification, or nutrification, is the addition of pure synthetic substances to foods in an attempt to put back what's been removed. And it's not only processing that destroys nutrients. From the moment plants are harvested, eggs are gathered, milk is collected, or livestock is slaughtered, there is an inevitable and progressive loss of the nutrients we need. Preserving foods is a way of minimizing the loss, but some methods are better than others. Freezing and smoking are the least destructive; canning and sterilization are the most destructive.

The food itself doesn't disintegrate—protein, fats, and carbohydrates are all relatively stable unless there is spoilage. But the parts of food that our bodies require to prevent disease—fiber, minerals, phytochemicals, and vitamins—are lost during the preservation process. As discussed in Chapter Three, when grains are milled, rice is polished, sugar is extracted, and oils and fats are separated, all the nutrients are removed as well. Many refined foods are so depleted of certain essential nutrients that the addition of pure chemically synthesized vitamins is required by law. One example is "enriched flour," which is used in all commercial breads.

Fortifying food is crucial in preventing disease. One of the biggest advances in nutritional science this century was the discovery that certain diseases were due to vitamin deficiencies in the diet. For instance, in the early twentieth century, pellagra—with symptoms such as mental deterioration, skin rashes, and diarrhea—was endemic in the southeastern United States, where the average diet was based on refined corn products. It was discovered that niacin was missing from the processed corn, and fortification began. Now that niacin is added to flour, breads, and grains, the disease is just about unheard of. Another example is goiter, a disease of the thyroid gland in which the gland becomes enlarged, resulting in hypothyroidism. Goiter is caused by insufficient iodine, and the problem has been just about eliminated with the addition of iodine to table salt. Now that synthetic vitamin D is added to milk, rickets, which used to cause bone deformities in children, has been eradicated. So it is possible to eliminate disease based on what we add to our food.

The homocysteine approach to heart disease says that deficiencies of vitamin B6, folic acid, and vitamin B12 are the underlying causes of arteriosclerosis and heart disease. Based on this idea, it would seem to be a simple matter to fortify refined foods with these vitamins to prevent the number one killer in this country—heart disease. So why hasn't this been done?

Federal Foodies: Who Decides on Fortification Levels

The job of the Food and Drug Administration is to assure the quality of the United States food supply. So part of the job of the FDA is to decide which foods should be fortified with which nutrients. The present policy authorizes fortification of foods according to the following principles:

(1) to conform with current food standards; (2) to replace nutrients at a level representative of those in the food prior to storage, handling, and processing; (3) to avoid nutritional inferiority in a food that replaces a traditional food in the diet [for example, to make sure that synthetic crabmeat has the same nutritional value as real crabmeat]; and (4) to balance the vitamin, mineral, and protein content of a food in proportion to its caloric content.

If the FDA doesn't mandate that a food be fortified, food manufacturers can voluntarily add vitamins, which is the case with breakfast cereals.

In making its decisions, the FDA considers the recommendations of the Food and Nutrition Board of the National

Research Council, which is responsible for determining the RDAs for each nutrient, as explained in Chapter Two. The FDA also considers the results of current surveys analyzing food consumption, such as the Nationwide Food Consumption Survey, the Continuing Survey of Food Intakes of Individuals, and the National Health and Nutrition Examination Surveys, all sponsored by the U.S. Department of Agriculture. Finally the FDA takes into account the opinions of nationally recognized experts in nutritional science.

This sounds like a lot of agencies and a lot of agendas— and that's exactly what it is. And that's what the problem is. The decision process is so complex that it happens at a glacial pace. On top of this, the FDA requires overwhelming scientific proof before it decides to fortify a food. This can take twenty-five to fifty years from the time a theory is published in scientific literature to when its importance has been proven conclusively in the population.

I'll give you an example of the byzantine nature of this process. In 1941 the decision was made to add four major nutrients—thiamin, riboflavin, niacin, and iron—to cereals, flour, and grain products. Today these three vitamins and one mineral are still used to fortify refined grain products. Sounds good so far. In 1974 the National Academy of Sciences and National Research Council proposed that this list be expanded to include pyridoxine, folic acid, vitamin A, calcium, magnesium, and zinc. Together with the original four, they are known as the Type 10 Formula. Whether these ten nutrients should be added to refined grain products was, and is still today, debated and analyzed. But, incredibly, the Type 10 Formula has never been implemented in the United States. These ten nutrients are not required to be added to refined foods even though it has been proven that they are depleted during processing. So the only required nutrients are the original four from 1941! In the meantime, the FDA has identified an expanded list of twenty-two nutrients—the Type 10 Formula plus twelve more—that are potential candidates for fortification of foods. Who knows? It may be another century before any action is taken on this list.

The Heart of the Matter: Fortification and Heart Disease

By now it should be clear from the first chapters of this book that processed foods are nutritionally empty. But the experts have known this for decades. The losses of vitamin B6 and folic acid during food processing have been clearly documented over the years. Nutrition surveys indicate that the average person in the United States consumes only 50 percent of the RDA for folic acid and 60 percent of the RDA for vitamin B6. And I don't think that the current RDA for B6 is even high enough.

Even though I formulated and proposed the homocysteine theory of heart disease twenty-five years ago, the nutrition establishment has refused to acknowledge the connection between vitamin deficiencies and heart disease. Adding folic acid and vitamin B6 to the food supply by fortification has not been taken seriously by the FDA. Now that the homocysteine theory has been proven in population studies, we can all hope that the FDA will start to consider seriously the fortification of foods with B6 and folic acid. So how much folic acid and B6 should we be getting? The results of the Health Canada Study and the Nurses Health Study have provided valuable information about the amounts we need to prevent heart disease. These studies say we should get 3 milligrams per day of vitamin B6 to minimize death from heart disease.

Luckily the RDA for folic acid has been increased to 400 micrograms per day. The recommendation of 400 micrograms was standard before 1989. It was then reduced to 200, partly because so few of the population were consuming the RDA of 400. Fortunately, the RDA for folic acid has been reinstated as 400 micrograms in the 1998 edition of Recommended Dietary Allowances. I say "luckily" because protection against heart disease is not the reason the decision was made—it's a side benefit.

After many hearings and many debates, the FDA finally decided to fortify cereal grain products with a small amount of folic acid, 140 micrograms per 100 grams. The RDA for folic acid was increased because it has been proven that folic acid helps prevent neural tube defects, a form of birth defects in newborns. This discovery was made twenty-five years ago, and controlled trials in the 1990s proved the connection beyond any doubt. Now you can see how long these actions take. But the FDA, in its decision to fortify cereal grain products with folic acid, did not mention folic acid lowering homocysteine levels and preventing heart disease. If it had, perhaps it would have considered increasing the level of fortification. As the new rules stand, the low level of added folic acid is still inadequate for the average person, and is certainly too little to help most of us achieve the 400 micrograms RDA.

In the case of vitamin B6, however, the new RDA levels are 1.3 to 1.7 milligrams per day for men and 1.3 to 1.5 milligrams per day for women. That's less than half the amount of B6 needed to counteract heart disease. So the first step is to set realistic RDAs. Then we have to fortify the food supply accordingly so that we can prevent heart disease.

When Food Fortification Works

Since the mid-1960s, deaths from heart disease have declined dramatically in the United States. The incidence today is less than one-half of what it was three decades ago. The National Institutes of Health held a conference to examine the possible reasons for this major decline. Their conclusion? None of the factors they looked at could account for more than a small fraction of the decline. For example, in the past thirty years blood cholesterol levels have been almost constant, declining only slightly (about 5 percent)—not enough to explain the major decline in heart disease deaths. Similarly, the amount of fat we're eating has increased slightly, so it's not the low-fat diet that's working. Other factors, such as stopping smoking, exercise, and improved surgical and medical therapy were considered to explain only a small part of this major decline.

But there isn't really a mystery here. The decline in heart disease deaths corresponds to the time when B6 consumption began to increase. About twenty years ago food manufacturers started voluntarily fortifying breakfast cereals with B6—even though the FDA didn't mandate it. Also, by the 1970s, many more people began taking vitamin supplements, increasing the average daily intake of B6 to more than 1 milligram per day per person. In the early 1980s the same thing happened with folic acid. So you can see that the addition of vitamin B6 and folic acid to the U.S. food supply explains the dramatic decline in deaths from heart disease since the 1960s.

Also since that time, we've been eating a lot more foods that contain the right vitamins. Because of improvements in transportation and distribution, fresh produce is now available all year throughout the country.

This solved mystery linking the decline in heart disease deaths to vitamin B supplementation shows us the power of food fortification. That's why we should make fortification mandatory. The current level of folic acid fortification could be tripled very safely to assure that every person in the United States would consume 400 micrograms per day of this vitamin.

So why aren't we doing that? In addition to the lengthy decision-making process, there is a persistent argument against this level of fortification. Some scientists say that a high level of folate in our bodies can mask the symptoms of a vitamin B12 deficiency—a deficiency that results either from a disease called pernicious anemia or from malabsorption. This could theoretically happen—some of the neurological effects of a severe deficiency could be exacerbated by folic acid. What these scientists don't mention is that this situation is extremely rare. In forty years of medical practice, I have never personally seen such a case. Furthermore, adequate vitamin B12 could be supplied by fortification and supplements to cover the bases.

The argument against fortifying foods with B6 is the theoretical risk of toxicity. In a total of seven known cases of toxicity, huge doses of B6 in the range of 1 to 6 grams per day were taken for months—*that's 1,000 to 3,000 times the RDA.* These seven people showed mild damage to their sensory nerves—neuropathy—as a result. In studies where high doses of B6 have been tested, toxicity wasn't a problem. In tests that study the effect of B6 on carpal tunnel syndrome, patients have received moderately large doses (up to 100 times the RDA) of the vitamin for years. In treatments of thousands of individuals with these doses of B6, not one single case of neuropathy developed in thirty years! One individual did develop a case of photosensitivity, which cleared up immediately when the dose of B6 was lowered.

So, overall, I don't think we're using fortification the way we should. The rare problem cases are scaring off the Food and Nutrition Board from implementing mandates that could save hundreds of thousands of lives—every year. Right now B6 is only added voluntarily, in cereals and by people taking supplements. Similarly, vitamin B12 is only added to a few foods voluntarily. And the new requirement for folic acid in cereal grain products is at an inadequate level. I believe that if we fortify refined foods with enough B6, folic acid, and B12, the deaths from heart disease would continue to decline—*at a much greater rate*. Vitamin B6 should be in enriched flour, cereal products, and other refined foods so that the average person gets a total of 3 milligrams per day. Similarly, the amount of folic acid added to flour and grain products should be increased so that everyone consumes 400 micrograms per day. And for those worried about the incredibly rare situation of a B12 deficiency being exacerbated, foods could be fortified with B12 to prevent it.

Should I or Shouldn't I? Vitamin Supplements

Fortifying foods is a way for the whole population to get the right vitamins. It's a public health measure that's designed to prevent disease. Because of our worries about the quality of fast food, and because we generally like to take matters into our own hands, a large portion of the U.S. population takes vitamins, minerals, or other dietary supplements.

It's not so easy figuring out exactly what to take. Every day the media subject us to a barrage of information about the health benefits of this or that pill. Just consider how many stories about vitamins you may have heard in the past year: supplements to combat osteoporosis, heart disease, cancer, arthritis; the list goes on. It seems we have an insatiable hunger for this kind of news—health in a pill.

If you decide to take supplements, choose the ones that you aren't getting enough of through the food you eat. If you are a meat-eater you should increase your intake of fruits and vegetables, and eliminate processed foods from your diet. During your transition to the Heart Revolution diet, to keep your blood homocysteine level low, consider taking folic acid and B6 supplements too. For strict vegetarians, a B12 supplement is a good idea. If you take a lot of medications, you should take a multivitamin that contains all three because many drugs antagonize the beneficial effects of these vitamins in your body. And think long-term. Vitamins may give you more energy, or ward off colds, but the real reason to take them is to prevent serious diseases down the road.

Should everyone take supplements, just to be safe? The truth is that if you are eating the Heart Revolution diet, with all the leafy green vegetables and fruits, *you don't need to take vitamins*.

For most Americans, that's a pretty big "if." But if you're truly concerned about your health, you will probably do whatever it takes to eat a good diet. As a start, read food labels, and eliminate transfats and refined foods. But should you take supplements anyway, just in case? If you can be diligent about food choices as well, that's fine. But we sometimes take the supplements *instead* of paying attention to our food. Popping a multivitamin with your Big Mac won't solve the problem. The whole foods that contain vitamins also have thousands of other beneficial compounds our bodies need, like phytochemicals, minerals, and fiber. Dietary supplements are highly purified or chemically synthesized compounds that have been proven to be active in the body. They don't have all the other nutrients that food contains. So if you're taking B vitamins as a safety net, don't forfeit eating well. I still believe that eating an optimal diet is the best way to maintain health and prevent disease.

Health for Sale: Choosing the Right Supplement

If you're young (below the magic age of forty), healthy, and eating the Heart Revolution diet, you don't need anything else. But the reality is that few people eat such a good diet. If you've been eating a poor-quality diet—lots of refined, packaged, and processed foods—or if you have early signs of arteriosclerosis and heart disease, supplements are a proven way to lower your blood homocysteine level. It is unreasonable to expect, however, that dietary supplements alone, without improving your diet, stopping smoking, exercising moderately, and controlling other risk factors, can reverse arteriosclerosis completely and restore arteries to perfect health. They're effective, but they can't work miracles.

If you have a family history of heart disease, this may be an indication that high homocysteine runs in your family. Or if you are obese, have high blood pressure, smoke, have diabetes, have elevated LDL or depressed HDL, or have early symptoms of arteriosclerosis, such as angina pectoris (chest pain), ischemic attacks (mini-strokes), or muscle pain when walking, you should have your doctor do a blood test to determine your homocysteine level. As for supplements, if your homocysteine level is below 8, you don't need to take B vitamins. If your homocysteine is around 10, you may have a mild B vitamin deficiency that can be corrected with about 3 milligrams per day of B6 and 400 micrograms per day of folic acid in the diet. That means eating lots of bananas, beans, whole grains, and fresh meats. If your homocysteine is above 15 or if you have carpal tunnel syndrome, you may have a greater deficiency of B6 or folic acid. Supplements of about 10–25 milligrams per day of B6 and 1 milligram of folic acid should bring it back to normal. A homocysteine of over 20 either indicates a serious nutritional deficiency or another severe condition, such as kidney failure. Talk to your doctor about such a possibility. If it's a nutritional deficiency, larger amounts in the range of 50–200 milligrams of B6 are needed. These doses of vitamin B6, more than you would find in an average multivitamin, have been proven safe when taken for years. In one study conducted in 1995, when these amounts were given, the risk of angina and heart attack was reduced by 75 percent. So if you have these symptoms, you can expect them to improve if you increase your B6 intake.

Folic acid is also an extremely safe vitamin to take in large doses. Even huge doses in animals have no toxic effects. Sometimes cancer patients who've had chemotherapy are given large amounts of folic acid because the chemotherapy drugs interfere with the action of folic acid. And again, if you read about folic acid masking neurological symptoms of a

B12 deficiency, this is an extremely rare situation and easily avoided by taking B12.

The amount of folic acid in most vitamin supplements, 400 micrograms, works so well that it lowers blood homocysteine levels in a week or two. Even if the homocysteine level is normal (5–10) folic acid will further decrease it by a small amount (1). There is no danger in having a very low homocysteine level.

Vitamin B12 is the one nutrient that we easily get enough of in our food. But as we get older, our bodies don't absorb it as well, so it's a good idea to take supplements if you're over sixty or a strict vegetarian. B12 becomes more difficult to absorb because about 10–15 percent of the population produces less of the protein called intrinsic factor in the stomach with age. Only about 1–2 percent of the vitamin B12 ingested can be absorbed without this intrinsic factor. There are several ways to solve this problem. First, the vitamin can be given by injection. This method is usually reserved for those with pernicious anemia, for the elderly who also have an inflamed stomach, or for vegans who eat no B12 from meat or dairy foods. Second, the vitamin can be placed under the tongue, so that more B12 is absorbed through the lining membrane of the mouth. Third, supplements containing 200–500 micrograms of the vitamin are available, so that even without the help of intrinsic factor, the average person will still get about 2–10 micrograms per day. If you've ever seen "antihomocysteine" multivitamins in the drugstore, they are loaded with 200–500 micrograms of B12. Vitamin B12 is also exceedingly safe to take, even in large doses; no toxic effects have ever been reported. Most multivitamins contain about 10 micrograms of B12, which is plenty.

If you're over the age of sixty to sixty-five, it makes sense to take an ordinary daily multivitamin to compensate for the decreased ability to absorb vitamins that happens as you age. To prevent heart disease, the supplement should contain 5–10 milligrams of vitamin B6, 400–1,000 micrograms of folic acid, and 200–1,000 micrograms of vitamin B12, in addition to 200–400 International Units (IU) of vitamin E, 60–200 milligrams of vitamin C, and balanced bulk and trace minerals. Some good nationally available brands are Twin Labs, Solgar, Centrum, Carlson, Sundown, and Theragran.

If you already have early symptoms of arteriosclerosis or severe conditions, like multiple heart attacks or strokes, kidney failure, diabetes, or hypothyroidism, you need a thorough evaluation by a competent physician. He or she can then help you to decide on the appropriate medical, dietary, lifestyle, and supplement strategy.

Increasingly, doctors are becoming aware of the need for homocysteine blood tests, especially in those with family histories of heart disease. In the future homocysteine testing should be a part of the standard testing for heart disease risk. In 1998 a new homocysteine test was made available for use in clinics and hospitals throughout the country to facilitate routine testing.

Suggested Supplements to Control Homocysteine

Disease Risk	Characteristics	Plasma Homocysteine (Micromoles per liter)	Supplements
Low	On Health Revolution diet	4–8	no supplements
Mild	Poor diet, over 60	8–12	3 mg B6 100 mg B12 400 mcg folic acid
Moderate	Poor diet, sedentary, obese, smoker, over 60	10–14	10 mg B6 100 mg B12 1,000 mcg folic acid
High	Family history, obesity, smoker, hypertension, high LDL, low HDL	12–20	50 mg B6 500 mg B12 2,000 mcg folic acid
Very high	Angina, ischemic attacks, kidney failure, diabetes	16–30	100 mg B6 1,000 mg B12 5,000 mcg folic acid

In addition to vitamin B6, vitamin B12, and folic acid, taking vitamin E, vitamin C and balanced bulk and trace minerals is also advisable to prevent heart disease.

6

Food Additives, Drugs, Alcohol, Smoking, Caffeine, and Hormones

When it comes to food, we get more than we pay for. In fact, there are so many foreign substances added to our food that sometimes what we think we're eating is only a small percentage of what's inside the package. If you look at a pint container of premium frozen yogurt, the last ingredient listed is yogurt culture. On all labels, ingredients are listed in descending order of percent composition, so when sugar is listed first on the frozen yogurt package, that means sugar is the primary ingredient.

We've all had the experience of looking at the long chemical names such as gluconolactone, carrageenan, sodium tripolyphosphate, gum arabic, potassium metabisulfite, sorbic acid, and glyceryl monolaurate listed as ingredients and wondering if we were actually eating food or plastic. These chemicals are usually preservatives that make food last longer or additives that enhance the flavor, texture, or color. Many of these ingredients are helpful—for example, BHA (butylated hydroxyanisole) and BHT (butylated hydroxytoluene) are added to preserve freshness. But as you might have guessed, not all of these chemicals are good for us.

What's in Our Food?
Food Additives and Preservatives

Chemical additives were developed in the nineteenth and early twentieth centuries for economic and practical reasons. Lower-cost elements were added to more expensive ingredients to expand the volume of the food or extend its shelf life. Sometimes they enhanced the color and flavor of poorly preserved foods. For example, at one time milk was diluted with water, chalk, starch, gums, or baking soda. Roasted carrots, beans, peas, and baked horse liver were added to coffee; other leaves were added to tea; sand, dust, lime, and pulp were added to sugar; water, salt, potato flour, and curds were added to butter; and alum and nonwheat flours were put in bread. At least these items were nontoxic. Other additives were much more dangerous: Lead or mercury salts laced beer, wine, and spices; turpentine oils were combined with olive oil or cod liver oil; and colorants that contained lead and arsenic were put into a variety of prepared foods. Can you imagine eating lead, arsenic, and turpentine?

The food supply just wasn't safe. For example, in the late nineteenth century, it wasn't unusual for commonly eaten foods prepared with lead salts to produce lead poisoning in children. Lead poisoning results in abdominal pain, anemia, and brain damage. So the Pure Food and Drug Act of 1906 was passed to regulate the purity and efficacy of foods and drugs, and the Food and Drug Administration became the governmental agency responsible for controlling adulteration of foods and regulating the practices of food manufacturers. Today we know much more about the chemical constituents of foods and just how toxic additives, preservatives, and contaminants can be. It's the FDA's responsibility to deal with all this information in carrying out its mandate to ensure the safety of our food supply.

The major offenders, such as lead, arsenic, and mercury salts, were eliminated from the food supply. These toxicants slowly damage liver, bone marrow, kidney, brain, and other tissues and can even kill you. Mercury causes brain damage (the phrase "mad as a hatter" comes from nineteenth-century England, where many hat makers suffered brain damage because of the mercury salts used in the industry. Some also say Isaac Newton died of mercury poisoning because of the mercury he used in certain experiments.) Other substances believed to have toxic effects over time, such as herbicides, pesticides, and hormones, have been controlled or eliminated if they're suspected of causing cancer or birth defects. Today, if a substance causes harmful effects in animal testing, it's eliminated. One example is red dye #2, which until 1990 was widely used in candy, Popsicles, and juices. When this dye showed evidence of producing cancer in lab rats, its use was discontinued.

However, a large number of other additives are used in foods not only to enhance flavor but also to stop microorganisms from growing. They are under the category known as

"Generally Recognized as Safe" (GRAS). Through the years, they haven't caused any serious harm, so they are considered safe. These additives have never been studied completely, so we don't know what they do to B vitamins.

Over the years, some things that we thought were safe turned out not to be so. Potassium nitrite stops molds and yeasts from growing and helps preserve and color meats. But nitrites have been shown to combine with chemicals in some foods, such as bacon, to produce carcinogens.

The FDA has quite a job, tracking and evaluating the effects of all possible additives. There are many complex chemical reactions that could occur. Because they can't possibly test every additive with every element in our bodies, we end up still eating processed, preserved, and packaged foods with additives that could potentially be harmful.

How do additives relate to homocysteine? If an additive interferes with B6, B12, or folic acid, homocysteine could rise. But to find this out, the FDA would have to test every possible additive to see its effect on these three vitamins. So far, this hasn't happened. So, in most instances, we don't know what the effects of chemical additives, preservatives, and contaminants on these sensitive B vitamins are. I recommend that the FDA test the effects of additives on these vitamins so we know what else contributes to high homocysteine levels.

I also know this is not easily accomplished. For example, a big effort has gone into evaluating food additives and contaminants to see what causes cancer in animals. But the FDA can't possibly test every additive. Nearly 3,000 substances are intentionally added to different foods during processing and preservation. About another 12,000 chemicals can contaminate foods through the packaging. While the FDA bans chemicals that test positive as carcinogenic, they can't test 15,000 substances with every element of our bodies. So for the vast majority of these additives and contaminants, we have too little information about whether they can cause cancer in experimental animals, never mind what they do to B vitamins. That's why it's so important to stick to fresh whole foods of the Heart Revolution diet.

Even less is known about these chemicals possibly causing cancer in humans. To make things even more complicated, there are naturally occurring carcinogens in some foods, such as aflatoxin of peanut molds, hydrazines of mushrooms, bracken fern toxins, plant tannins, safrole from saffron, and urethane from fermented foods. Minute quantities of these carcinogens have been found in plant foods, seasonings, beer, and wine. Eating the phytochemicals and other nutrients in the Heart Revolution diet helps to counteract and prevent the effects of these naturally occurring carcinogens.

Some preservatives work against chemical carcinogens and can actually protect us from cancer. BHA and BHT prevent fats in food from reacting with oxygen, and so retard spoilage. This same property also helps to protect against stomach cancer in humans. Other widely used additives include thickeners and stabilizers, flavor enhancers, emulsifiers, acidulants, chemical leavening agents, colorants, humectants (moisteners), nutritional supplements, preservatives, enzymes, nonnutritive sweeteners, sugar, and antioxidants. In most cases the effects of these many additives on B6, folic acid, and B12 are simply unknown.

Foods have been preserved by smoke for thousands of years. But smoke contains chemical carcinogens that have been found to cause stomach cancer in people in Iceland

and Japan. The point is that some additives help, and others are really quite dangerous. But no one knows just how each one affects folic acid and B6 in foods or in the body. There could be hundreds of added chemicals that interfere with the body's ability to function normally. Is it worth taking the risk and eating all these foreign substances when you don't have to?

Synthetic Foods: Olestra and Transfats

What about the chemical substances that imitate food? Who wouldn't want to save a few calories by using a fat substitute? Well, it depends on whom you talk to. The food industry has spent quite a lot of time and money developing synthetic fat-like substances such as olestra (Olean is the brand name of olestra). These additives were designed to give a fatlike consistency and flavor to low-fat foods. And they do. But fake fat is not absorbed from the intestine; instead, it's simply excreted, taking vitamins A, E, and D, as well as essential oils and ubiquinone along with it. While olestra doesn't add calories, it doesn't add nutrients, either. But worst of all, it actually decreases the body's ability to absorb vitamins from other foods. Fake fats were created in response to our fear of fat, which is partly due to the faulty cholesterol theory of heart disease. They may save a few calories, but from a health perspective, they are quite damaging, and I would avoid them at all costs.

The dangers of chemically altered fats—transfats from hydrogenated oils, margarine, and shortening—have been described earlier in the book. Like synthetic fats, these hydrogenated oils should never be eaten. It's easy to avoid them once you're in the habit of reading the list of ingredients on food labels. The transfats of hydrogenated oils have been proven to increase the risk of arteriosclerosis and heart disease. Why take that risk?

Finding Safe Food: Shopping for Food

The food supply in the United States is incredibly safe, especially compared to that of other countries. But the effort of food inspectors, producers, preparers, and marketers can't let up, in fact it should increase. The outbreaks of food contamination in the past few years from *E. coli O157:H7*, *Salmonella*, *Shigella*, *Campylobacter*, *Cyclospora*, *Yersinia*, and *Listeria* are warnings that we constantly have to protect the safety of our food supply. The old threats don't disappear, such as shellfish contaminated with viruses like hepatitis A, chickens and eggs tainted with *Salmonella*, seafood infested with *Vibrio cholerae*, and canned goods filled with *Clostridium botulinum*. Newer threats are protozoa like *Cryptosporidium*, *Giardia*, and *Cyclospora* that get into our water supply; bovine spongioform encephalopathy (mad cow disease) from cattle fed animal residue; and *Listeria* from milk, cheese, and poorly washed vegetables.

Pathogenic microorganisms enter the food supply by a variety of routes. Animals may be fed diets that encourage overgrowth of pathogenic microorganisms. In 1998 the feeding of hay to cattle was found to decrease the risk of *E. coli* contamination originally produced by feeding grains to cattle. Overall, the more mechanized and automated the production of foods, the more these threats will recur in the future. Machines break down and bacteria can get into the food supply. In some cases, contaminants have originated from poor personal hygiene, hence the signs for handwashing in restaurant bathrooms.

All we have to do to avoid contamination is select the freshest possible produce, meats, fish, and dairy foods, then wash and cook foods thoroughly, and refrigerate or freeze any leftovers right away. (It's actually better to toss out all leftovers, but some people just can't bear to part with them.) Foods that are grown on local farms may be the least likely to be contaminated if the farm is clean and the workers observe proper hygiene. And because the food is fresh, the B6, folic acid, and B12 don't have a chance to degenerate.

Admittedly, the more we know about nutrition, the more difficult food shopping becomes. This is ironic, because the idea here is to eat the simplest, freshest whole foods, just like our hunter-gatherer ancestors did. But sometimes getting back to basics is the hardest thing to do. So when you're in the supermarket looking for the healthiest whole foods, how do you know what they are?

Consider organic food. Theoretically it's cultivated and harvested without the use of pesticides, hormones, antibiotics, or chemical fertilizers, relying instead on natural fertilizers, biological pest control, and minimum tillage cultivation. As a result, many people prefer organic foods because they contain fewer chemicals. At present there are few regulations assuring these practices, so it's hard to know if food labeled "organic" is actually better. In terms of homocysteine, there is no evidence that the content of folic acid and vitamin B6 is greater in organic foods.

I've been lucky that supermarkets in my area carry traditionally produced crops, not labeled "organic," that are generally of excellent quality and have as many vitamins, minerals, and other nutrients as organic foods. Of course, the best way to buy vegetables is at a local farm stand, where the time from picking to purchasing is the shortest.

Hydroponic foods are another good choice. These are usually found in little plastic containers in the produce section. This type of cultivation uses only mineral solutions and water to grow vegetables such as lettuce. With sunlight, air, and temperature control, plants can make all their tissues without soil. An advantage of hydroponic agriculture over other methods is that it's rigorously controlled, so the vegetables shouldn't contain any pesticide residues or other contaminants.

One last note about fresh food: In Chapter Three I talked about irradiation as a way to sterilize food. The food industry has advocated using this method to combat contamination by microorganisms. But there is a serious problem with irradiating food. The sensitive vitamins, folic acid and vitamin B6, are partially destroyed by the radiation just as they are by canning and sterilization. Technology, in its attempt to protect us, is actually harming our food supply. The farther away we get from simple, whole foods, the less beneficial our food becomes.

Hello Dolly: Genetic Engineering

In recent years, cross-bred vegetables have been in vogue, especially in cities and fashionable restaurants. Some are designed to be "cancer-fighting" vegetables since they've been created with enhanced phytochemical properties. But a lot of what we eat is genetically modified, even if it doesn't get the same press. In 1998 the government gave the green light to genetically altered soybeans, cotton, corn, summer squash, potatoes, canola oil, radicchio, papayas, and tomatoes. Today 32 percent of the soybean crop has been genetically manipulated.

The idea of genetically engineered food isn't new. For centuries plants and animals have been selected and bred to yield better food. You remember Dolly, the cloned sheep, and the dozens of cloned mice created in 1998. While cloning is now getting headlines, it has long been used to create superior vines for the production of high-quality grapes and wine. Perhaps through some of these new methods, scientists can create foods that provide the B6 and folic acid we need to prevent heart disease.

Altered States: Drugs, Homocysteine, and Heart Disease

Fortunately, it hasn't been shown that most common drugs affect homocysteine levels in the body. But it's worth discussing the few drugs that have known effects on homocysteine. In any case, it is never advisable to stop medication without consulting your doctor.

It's no surprise that drugs can have an enormous effect on the delicate chemical balance in our bodies, which is why we take them in the first place. But if a drug prevents B6, folic acid, or B12 from doing their jobs, homocysteine levels will rise.

One such drug is methotrexate, commonly used in cancer chemotherapy. Methotrexate, the first widely used chemotherapeutic drug for treating childhood leukemia, causes blood homocysteine levels to rise within hours after administration.

But methotrexate interferes with folic acid in the body, and so homocysteine levels rise. So far, its benefits in treating cancer have greatly outweighed the risk of high homocysteine's damaging arteries, especially since children are at a low risk of arteriosclerosis anyway because of their generally low homocysteine levels.

Laughing gas (nitrous oxide) is another drug that affects homocysteine in the blood. This gas causes blood homocysteine to rise quickly because it interferes with vitamin B12 within cells and tissues. The effect is temporary, and therefore it probably damages arteries only minimally. Of course, we don't know what happens to dentists and anesthesiologists who are exposed to low levels of the gas more frequently. A recent experiment showed that pigs exposed to nitrous oxide had not only high homocysteine levels but significant damage to their hearts. Next time you're at the dentist, Novocain might be the better choice. However, if you're allergic to Novocain or you're at high risk of heart disease, it may be worth supplementing your diet with B vitamins during prolonged dental work if nitrous oxide is being used for anesthesia.

Azaribine, a toxic drug used to fight certain cancers, also causes homocysteine to rise. Because of its extreme toxicity, the drug was not widely used after its discovery in the 1950s. But in the 1970s azaribine was given to suppress cell growth in patients with refractory psoriasis, a chronic skin disease usually treated with coal tar and ultraviolet light. Within a few years patients taking the drug for psoriasis experienced heart attack, stroke, and thrombosis. It was then determined that azaribine prevented B6 from acting in the body, and homocysteine levels shot through the roof, as did vascular disease. For this reason, in 1977, the FDA recalled azaribine for use in psoriasis, the first such recall of any FDA-approved drug in the history of the agency.

Even commonly prescribed drugs have been found to cause homocysteine levels to rise. One example is phenytoin (Dilantin), which controls epileptic seizures. This drug antagonizes folic acid and causes homocysteine levels to rise slightly, potentially causing damage to arteries over a period of years. Other anticonvulsant drugs—phenobarbital, primidone, carbamazepine, and valproic acid—also cause a deficiency of folic acid, and so homocysteine levels go up. Some diuretic drugs (thiazides) prescribed to lower blood pressure cause homocysteine to rise.

If you are on any of these drugs, you should err on the safe side and take folic acid and B vitamin supplements.

The Lowdown on Statin: Cholesterol-Lowering Drugs

We've all seen the ads in the newspapers and on TV, or perhaps you or someone you know is taking a cholesterol-lowering drug. These drugs would seem to be the perfect way to prevent or cure heart disease—assuming it was caused only by high cholesterol. Within the past few years these "statin" drugs—lovastatin, pravastatin, simvistatin, and fluvastatin—have become enormously popular. They work by decreasing the production of cholesterol by the liver.

But again, I want to make it clear that the cholesterol is not the primary cause of heart disease. It only exacerbates the situation once the damage has been done by homocysteine. Lowering cholesterol can help if you already have heart disease. But because these drugs lower LDL, they do tend to decrease the risk of heart disease for those in high-risk groups.

LDL carries homocysteine to artery walls where plaques are produced. In lowering LDL (and keeping homocysteine away from arteries), statin drugs can prevent an already bad situation from getting any worse.

But there are some very serious, major complications associated with these drugs that you will never hear about in the ads or read in the fine print. First of all, they decrease the production of ubiquinone (coenzyme Q10), which can weaken the heart muscle and make it more likely to fail. Within the past decade, the use of statin drugs has greatly increased. While the deaths from heart disease and heart attack have declined, the incidence of death from heart *failure* has *increased* in the past fifteen years. We're not sure if the increase in these drugs is directly related to the increase in deaths due to heart failure, but this certainly warrants more scrutiny. Coenzyme Q10, made in the body, derived from meats and nuts, and available in supplement form at health food stores, should definitely be taken by anyone on statin drugs to make sure the heart is not affected in this way.

Secondly, statins can cause severe side effects. Many patients taking statin drugs have evidence of liver toxicity and gastrointestinal side effects such as bloating and diarrhea. Liver toxicity causes abnormal liver function and may cause jaundice in extreme cases. In a few, fortunately rare, cases the statin drugs are responsible for devastating damage to muscles, causing severe weakness throughout the body.

The most alarming news is that all the statin drugs *have been proven to cause cancer in laboratory animals*. There is a very real risk of cancer in people using these drugs as well. For this reason, experts have recommended that the statin drugs be used only in people with a short life expectancy—five to ten years. However, the proponents of statin drug therapy and certain pharmaceutical companies have suggested prescribing these toxic drugs to obese children who are at risk of developing heart disease in adulthood. Because of the dangers of statin drugs, I believe it is unacceptable to prescribe them to children.

I recommend that these potent drugs should be used only if you have very high cholesterol levels (over 300) and reduced life expectancy because of heart disease. Isn't it easier just to eat right, maybe take a daily B6, B12, and folic acid supplement?

"Legal" Drugs: Alcohol, Smoking, and Caffeine

Alcohol

I hope that by now you are more aware of what you're eating, are avoiding refined carbohydrates, are loading up on vegetables, are scanning labels for hydrogenated oils, and are staying away from packaged, preserved foods. But what about alcohol? I'm sure you've heard the news that drinking moderate amounts of red wine is actually good for your heart. Now I'm going to tell you why.

Alcohol has been around since the Agricultural Revolution 10,000 years ago. Cultivated and wild grapes were fermented and made into alcohol by Neolithic man. The ancient Greek and Roman civilizations depended on vineyards and wine production for trade and commerce. Once grains were cultivated, beer making soon followed, as did distillation of spirits from both grapes and grains.

The health benefits of wine have actually been known since the nineteenth century. And in fact, studies show that those who don't drink any alcohol have a slightly shorter life expectancy than moderate consumers. (Of course, alcohol abusers die younger because of accidents, cirrhosis of the liver, brain toxicity, and other complications.) Many studies have documented the benefits of alcohol in relation to heart disease. Most research indicates that the skins of the grapes contain phytochemicals that protect the heart. These substances may be partly responsible for the so-called French paradox, which refers to the low incidence of heart disease among the French despite their relatively rich diets. Since the French drink red wine frequently, these antioxidants are protecting their hearts. In addition, the modest amount of vitamin B6 and folic acid in wine helps to prevent elevated homocysteine levels. But the French also eat a lot of B vitamins and little processed or refined foods, so their homocysteine is kept low that way as well.

Wine, a natural product made from grape juice, contains alcohol when allowed to ferment with yeast. While the stems and other debris are removed before bottling, all of the grapes' minerals and phytochemicals, as well as some of the vitamins, stay in the final product. Sulfites are added to most wines as a preservative. Red wine contains healthful pigments (polyphenol antioxidants and tannins) from the grape skins; so does white wine, but in lesser amounts. Because of the high concentration of pigments, red is a better choice.

Hard liquors—whiskey, brandy, gin, rum, and grain alcohol—are all severely depleted in minerals, vitamins, and phytochemicals. People who abuse hard liquor tend to become deficient in folic acid, thiamin, and other vitamins. Chronic alcoholics often have high blood homocysteine as a result. On the other hand, if you drink any kind of alcohol only moderately (one to two drinks per day) and consume a lot of folic acid, you'll be less likely to die from heart disease.

Drinking beer can also lead to depletion of folic acid, thiamin, and other vitamins, and so homocysteine goes up. Heavy beer drinkers have a tendency to skip vitamin-rich foods, potentially leading to deficiencies. If you are going to drink, it is best to stick to moderate amounts of red wine (one to two glasses per day) consumed with meals. Skip beer and hard liquor.

Smoking

While drinking wine in moderation actually has benefits, there are absolutely no health benefits to smoking. Knowing the details may help this fact sink in. Although my father had ancestors with extraordinary longevity, he died of cancer at age fifty-nine because of a lifelong addiction to smoking. Cigarette smoke contains over 600 toxic compounds, many of which can cause cancer in humans and animals. Cigarette smoking is also a potent risk factor for heart disease. One of the major gases in cigarette smoke is carbon monoxide—the very same gas people use to commit suicide. This gas combines with hemoglobin in red blood cells and with other proteins and enzymes and prevents normal metabolism of oxygen within cells. Carbon monoxide also combines with a form of vitamin B6 (pyridoxamine) within the body to inactivate the vitamin. Cigarette smoking decreases the level of vitamin B6 and increases the level of homocysteine in the blood. This is how smoking causes heart attacks, arteriosclerosis of the peripheral arteries, and other vascular complications. It's that simple. And that deadly.

All tobacco products can have life-threatening consequences. Cigarettes, cigars, pipes, and chewing tobacco are responsible for the current epidemic of lung cancer, cancer of the mouth, cancer of the larynx, cancer of the kidney, and cancer of the bladder. Did you know that lung cancer in women causes more deaths than breast cancer, colon cancer, pancreatic cancer, skin cancer, or liver cancer? Burning tobacco releases tars and other combustion byproducts that contain highly carcinogenic free radical compounds. That's bad enough. But when these compounds interact with cells, they deplete a form of homocysteine (thioretinaco) from cell membranes, transforming normal cells into cancer cells. Smokers who abuse alcohol have a much greater risk of cancer of the mouth, esophagus, and larynx because the alcohol makes the effect of the carcinogens on cells even worse, as we understand it now. This in turn rapidly depletes the homocysteine compound from those cells, transforming them into cancer cells.

And that's only part of the story. All smokers suffer tremendous damage to their lungs because the carbon monoxide, among other things, destroys the lung's elastic tissues. If someone smokes over a period of years, this destructive effect leads to chronic infections, increased fibrous tissue, stiffness of the lung, and overexpansion of the lung. This severe lung damage is what's known as emphysema and chronic bronchitis, which are leading causes of death and disability among smokers. Now that you know about all these complications, you will be more conscious about the dangers of smoking. If you're improving what you eat, don't diminish your efforts by smoking.

Caffeine

On a lighter note, caffeine is another drug that most of us use pretty regularly. But even caffeine can be abused, and then it, too, affects homocysteine. If you're drinking large amounts of coffee (more than six cups per day) blood homocysteine rises slightly, about 1 micromole per liter, as shown by the Hordaland Homocysteine Study. Although a few studies have suggested that large amounts of coffee may contribute to risk of pancreatic cancer, most studies have concluded that moderate coffee drinking is safe. Many coffee drinkers add cream and sugar, but sugar should be eliminated when following the Heart Revolution diet.

Tea, which contains less caffeine than coffee, has no effect on homocysteine. It's a safer option for those worried about homocysteine. By now you've probably heard about green tea, which is being put into everything from ice cream to skin creams. Green tea and herbal teas are the least damaging of all, and can have beneficial effects. Green tea actually tastes pretty good and has a little caffeine in it, too, so you can have the best of both worlds.

Circuit Breakers: Hormones and Homocysteine

By now most of us know that men are more susceptible to heart disease and arteriosclerosis than women. But a woman's risk of heart disease increases rapidly after menopause, when her susceptibility equals that of a man. Heart disease actually kills more women every year than breast cancer.

Some of the earliest studies of homocysteine and heart

disease showed that men have higher levels of homocysteine than do women of the same age. Generally the blood homocysteine levels of men are in the 8–12 micromoles per liter range, and women of the same age have levels of 6–10 micromoles per liter. This is why men are more susceptible to heart disease than women. After menopause, however, the homocysteine level in women rapidly increases to approach that of men, and so does the risk of heart disease. This is not a coincidence. The increased risk is a direct result of increased homocysteine levels.

Hormones have a large effect on controlling homocysteine. When the ovaries stop producing estrogen and progestin during menopause, homocysteine levels rise. Hormone replacement therapy in postmenopausal women causes homocysteine to go down moderately, generally in the range of 15 percent. It has been proven that postmenopausal women taking estrogen and progesterone therapy are partly protected against heart disease, and this decrease in homocysteine explains why.

Does this mean that women taking birth control pills have even greater protection against heart disease? In the 1950s, when oral contraceptives were first introduced, they contained high doses of estrogens and progestins. Within a few years women taking these pills were found to have a greater risk of thrombosis, embolism, and vascular damage than young women not on the pill. This would seem to contradict what I said before about the protective benefits of hormone replacement therapy. But it turns out that very high doses of these hormones inhibit the protective benefits of vitamin B6 and folic acid in the body. As a result, there is an abnormal amount of homocysteine in the blood. The original pill contained high doses of hormones; today's pill does not.

A delicate balance of female hormones is required to control homocysteine—too little, and homocysteine goes up; too much, and vitamin B6 and folic acid can't control homocysteine. That's why it's important to work with your doctor to determine the correct amount of estrogen to take. Hormone replacement therapy may be of additional benefit in women who are at increased risk of heart disease because of dietary, genetic, smoking, and other risk factors.

The vascular problems first associated with the pill have almost disappeared because the amount of estrogen and progesterone in oral contraceptives is so much lower now than when they were first introduced. But if you smoke while you are on the pill, there is definitely a slightly increased risk of thrombosis and embolism. This is because smoking, like contraceptive hormones, impairs the actions of vitamin B6 and folic acid in the body, causing homocysteine levels to rise.

For many years it has been known that a deficiency of thyroid hormone increases our chances of getting heart disease. Doctors long thought this was the result of an increase in blood cholesterol, triglycerides, and LDL. Not surprisingly, it's now been found that homocysteine also increases when there is too little thyroid hormone, accounting for the increase in risk of heart disease.

Counter to what you might think, when severe hypothyroidism is treated with large doses of thyroid hormone, the risk of heart attack is greatly increased during the first few days of treatment. This probably occurs because the thyroid hormone stimulates metabolism, stressing the heart. However, small doses of thyroid hormone gradually decrease the levels of homocysteine, and so the risk of heart disease is decreased over a period of years. So again, it's a delicate balance of how much thyroid hormone you need to function properly without affecting your risk of heart disease. If you are being treated for a thyroid condition, talk with your doctor about your homocysteine level, especially if you have a family history of heart disease.

Protective Drugs

Some drugs affect hormones, and consequently the risk of heart disease. In the past few years the drug tamoxifen, which affects estrogen, has not only been widely used to treat breast cancer, but has been prescribed to some women who are at a high risk for the disease. In clinical studies women who were taking the drug for breast cancer also had a significantly reduced risk of heart disease. Again, this is because of the effect on homocysteine; tamoxifen decreases homocysteine in the blood substantially, and so women taking it are protected against heart disease. Because of sometimes toxic side effects, however, the drug is not generally used in women unless they have or are at high risk for breast cancer or other forms of malignancy. But if you must take this potentially toxic drug, one benefit is that you will have protection from heart disease.

Hundreds of other substances, both outside and inside the body, may potentially affect homocysteine levels. Every day I receive two to three medical papers reporting on studies monitoring the effects of various substances on homocysteine. I hope that in the coming years we will have a much greater understanding of what it takes to keep homocysteine levels low.

Controlling Contaminants: Practical Tips

- Don't eat any packaged foods containing partially hydrogenated oils, synthetic fat substitutes, powdered eggs, or powdered milk. These products contain contaminants that increase the risk of heart disease.

- Avoid moldy peanuts; meats cured with nitrites, such as bologna, salami, and liverwurst; heavily salted and smoked foods; foods seasoned with large amounts of saffron; and large amounts of common mushrooms. They contain natural carcinogens that increase the risk of cancer.

- Buy vegetables produced on local farms in season or select the freshest produce shipped from other states and countries in the winter and early spring months. These foods contain the largest amounts of folic acid and vitamin B6.

- Don't eat anything preserved by irradiation, which reduces the amount of folic acid and vitamin B6 in foods.

- Use statin drugs to lower cholesterol levels only if after six months of eating the Heart Revolution diet and taking B vitamin supplements, homocysteine levels have not dropped to normal. These potent statin drugs should really only be taken by people with a short life expectancy because of their ability to cause cancer and other toxic effects.

- If you are taking statin drugs, supplement the therapy with coenzyme Q10.

- Consume a glass or two of red wine with meals several days per week.

- Try to avoid distilled liquors like gin, vodka, scotch, and whiskey since they're deficient in minerals, vitamins, and other essential nutrients. The large amount of alcohol in spirits can also cause toxic effects on the liver and brain.

- Limit beer consumption because of its high caloric content and chemical additives.

- Treat the need to stop smoking cigarettes, pipes, and cigars and using chewing tobacco as a medical emergency. These enormously destructive products cause addiction, disease, and shortened life span in children and adults who use them.

- Limit coffee consumption to one or two cups per day. Alternate coffee with tea, herbal tea, and green tea, which contain beneficial phytochemicals and less caffeine.

- Use only low-dose contraceptive hormones during the reproductive years, and never smoke while using these drugs.

- Consider the use of hormone replacement therapy after menopause if you have multiple risk factors for heart disease.

- Have your doctor check your thyroid function in cases where homocysteine elevation in the blood is unexplained. Untreated hypothyroidism increases the risk of heart disease.

7

Exercise and Obesity

Have you ever felt the difference between taking a walk after dinner and sitting, watching TV? Do you know the feeling of exhilaration when you ride a bike to the top of a hill, without having to walk it part of the way? How about finishing a walk-a-thon, running a five-kilometer race, swimming a mile, or even competing in a triathlon? Exercise has short-term feel-good benefits—the "thrill of victory"—and long-term health benefits—improving your quality of life, preventing disease, and maximizing your chance for a longer life.

Or does the idea of sweating make your teeth hurt? If so, you're not alone. Only about 15 percent of Americans exercise vigorously for at least twenty minutes, three times a week or more. And according to the 1996 report of the U.S. Surgeon General, *Physical Activity and Health*, over 60 percent of adults don't get enough physical activity, even moderate activity, and 25 percent don't get any activity at all. You've heard it before, but these figures show that Americans are sedentary.

There are some major consequences of our, shall we say, relaxed lifestyle. Inactivity and poor nutrition are right up there with smoking in terms of causes of death in the United States. Studies show that those who don't exercise die two to three years earlier than those who do. In one study the least fit men were one and a half times as likely to die prematurely as the men who were the most fit, and women in the low-fitness category were twice as likely to die early as women who were the most fit.

When it comes to heart disease, the numbers are staggering. Inactivity contributes to more than a third of the nearly 500,000 annual heart disease deaths a year, according to the U.S. Center for Disease Control and Prevention. If you don't exercise, you have twice as great a risk of getting heart disease as someone who exercises regularly. But if you are active, you have a 23 percent less chance of dying from heart disease. And if you exercise vigorously, the risk goes down even more. Overall, exercising vigorously at least three hours a week has been shown to reduce the chance of having a heart attack or stroke by 60 percent.

The good news is that increasing your activity level is probably the easiest thing to do, with the most dramatic results. In addition to helping prevent heart disease, physical activity has wide-ranging health benefits, including reducing the risk of certain cancers like colon cancer, diabetes, and osteoporosis. Exercise also lowers blood pressure, increases the good HDL cholesterol level, and fights obesity (which we'll get to later in the chapter), and has a positive effect on mental health.

Making the Connection: Homocysteine and Exercise

So how does exercise actually work in the body? On a simple level, when you exercise, your muscles work harder. Muscles need oxygen and energy to work, so there is an increased demand on your respiratory and circulatory systems. More blood gets pumped through your arteries and veins. The actual volume of blood in your body increases as well. The heart doesn't have to beat as fast because more blood is released with each contraction. The heart is pumping more efficiently, and so your resting blood pressure is lowered. You probably know that athletes have a much lower resting heart rate than couch potatoes.

The fats in the bloodstream change as well. Exercise reduces blood triglyceride levels, and high triglycerides in the blood have been linked to an increased risk of heart attack. What happens is that exercise makes the muscles hungry for fat, so the muscles increase the production of an enzyme called lipoprotein lipase (LPL), which chews up triglycerides for the muscles to use as fuel. If there is a weight loss due to regular exercise, the LPL activity in fat cells increases even more and so more triglycerides are used up, further reducing the risk of heart attack. The "good" cholesterol, HDL, also increases, which helps remove fatty deposits from artery walls.

So how does homocysteine fit in? A 1995 study of homo-cysteine and risk factors definitively showed that physical activity significantly lowers homocysteine levels. We've always known that exercise reduces our chance of getting heart disease, but no one could explain why. Now we know that exercise has a positive effect on homocysteine levels, cutting the risk of heart disease.

The greatest benefits of exercise—strength, endurance, and mental alertness—are seen in the oldest age groups. This means that it's never too late to start exercising, especially since your homocysteine level will go down as a result.

Why Cavemen Were More Fit Than We Are, and Why That Matters

Nothing seems more modern than a sleek health club, complete with large-screen TVs, headsets, music videos, and various cardio machines flashing the number of calories we're burning. But when you think about it, there is something a little barbaric about exercising in these cavernous gyms. What we're really doing is trying to imitate the exercise patterns of our ancestors, the hunter-gatherers. Not only did they have the ideal diet, but also they exercised—a lot. They had to.

Humans in prehistoric times would often spend a day or more tracking and hunting animals at a running or jogging pace. Then they would carry the animal back to camp—probably strapped to their backs—at a relatively fast clip, too. On their rest days when they were celebrating and feasting, they would still take walks—six to twenty miles—to visit relatives and friends.

Even when it was not a matter of finding food, shelter, or safety, prehistoric people were physically active. They enjoyed it. It was part of their social, religious, and cultural lives.

It has been estimated that hunter-gatherers used about 3,000 calories a day in energy expenditure. Although a construction worker today might expend 3,500 calories, the average adult burns only about 1,800–2,000 calories a day. The industrial and technological revolutions have made it easier to be sedentary. In the past hundred years, our physical activity rates have dropped dramatically. Even our grandparents burned 300–400 more calories than we do. We don't need to move around so much when there are conveyer belts, people-movers, cars, trains, and supermarkets, not to mention e-mail and telephones.

So who cares about the cavemen? Unfortunately, our bodies have not really changed much since prehistoric times. In terms of diet and exercise, evolution has not caught up with our modern lifestyles. Our bodies need exercise to stay healthy and prevent disease. We are evolved to move, but our society has conditioned us not to. But exercise can be incorporated into your daily life so that it seems completely natural. It should be natural because it is.

How Much Can We Get Away with Doing, or Not Doing?

One reason Americans don't exercise enough is our perception of exercise. People think it has to be flat-out exhausting to be worth the time, or that you have to be in shape to be able to exercise. This simply isn't true. In fact, the people who go from not exercising at all to moderate activity get the most health benefits. And no matter what you weigh, exercising will reduce your risk of disease and early death.

To drive home this point, the U.S. Center for Disease Control and Prevention (CDC), as well as lots of other health-related organizations, such as the American College of Sports Medicine and the National Institutes of Health, have made recommendations for moderate exercise that are supported by the U.S. Surgeon General. The idea is that moderate exercise is what you need to reduce the risk of disease and mortality.

So what's moderate? You can get by on thirty minutes of activity most days of the week. And the thirty minutes doesn't even have to be continuous. It can be ten minutes of gardening in the morning, a brisk walk at lunch, and then a ten-minute bike ride after dinner. The goal is to burn 150 calories a day in the form of exercise, or 1,000 calories a week, and thirty minutes a day of walking will do that.

Examples of Moderate Amounts of Physical Activities

In increasing order of exertion, each item listed represents 150 calories burned.

Washing and waxing a car for forty-five to sixty minutes
Washing windows or floors for forty-five to sixty minutes
Playing volleyball for forty-five minutes
Playing touch football for thirty to forty-five minutes
Gardening for thirty to forty-five minutes
Wheeling self in wheelchair for thirty to forty-five minutes
Walking one and three-quarter miles in thirty-five minutes (twenty minutes per mile)
Basketball (shooting baskets) for thirty minutes
Bicycling five miles in thirty minutes
Dancing fast (social) for thirty minutes
Pushing a stroller one and a half miles in thirty minutes

Raking leaves for thirty minutes

Walking two miles in thirty minutes (fifteen minutes per
   mile)

Water aerobics for thirty minutes

Swimming laps for twenty minutes

Wheelchair basketball for twenty minutes

Basketball (playing a game) for fifteen to twenty minutes

Bicycling four miles in fifteen minutes

Jumping rope for fifteen minutes

Running one and a half miles in fifteen minutes (ten
   minutes per mile)

Shoveling snow for fifteen minutes

Stairwalking for fifteen minutes

These recommendations created quite a stir in 1993 when
the CDC announced that only moderate activity was necessary to reap health benefits. It had previously recommended
thirty minutes of sustained aerobic exercise at least three
times a week. The new approach seemed so much easier. In
1996 the Surgeon General's report echoed the new idea of
"exercise-lite." Exercise shouldn't be intimidating, and if
thirty minutes a day of accumulated activity during the day
will enable you to live longer, then why not do it?

Of course, the more you do, the more health benefits you
get. The Nurses' Health Study showed that women who
walked at a slow pace had a 32 percent lower risk of heart
attack and stroke than those who were sedentary. Women
who walked briskly (three to four miles per hour) at least
three hours per week had a 54 percent lower risk. Another
study found that the chance of having a heart attack in the
next ten years was 30 percent lower for those who ran forty to
fifty miles a week than for those who ran less than ten miles a

week. Let's face it, how many of us can even dream of running that much? But the point is the more we exercise, the more benefits we get—up to a point. If you are an extreme exerciser, such as a marathoner, the added benefits from strenuous exercise not only taper off, but start to decrease.

Getting to Go

So everyone agrees that we need to exercise. Getting started is not as hard as you might think. The first step is to figure out what works best for you. I tried jogging when it first became popular in the seventies, but I didn't like it. I felt that it was too hard on my joints. Now I play tennis several times a week, take walks, and do plenty of yard work, including gardening, raking leaves, pruning hedges, and planting bushes. I could probably do more, but I know I am burning the 1,000 extra calories per week that the CDC suggests to get health benefits.

The key is to find your own rhythm so you'll stick with it. Many people buy home treadmills and walk uphill while watching the news on TV. Others have a walking partner and walk briskly every day, or every other day. One woman we know listens to books on tape while she walks. Try walking the golf course instead of riding in a cart, parking in the farthest spot from the office or mall, walking into town for the newspaper, taking the stairs instead of the elevator, playing actively with your kids or grandchildren, carrying the groceries to the car instead of pushing them in a cart, dancing, joining a tennis club, walking to a neighbor's dinner party instead of driving, planting a cutting garden, cleaning out the garage; anything that requires you to move more than you do now. You want to enjoy what you're doing as well, so you'll keep doing it.

A lot of people have a hard time believing that walking is optimal exercise. But it is. Brisk walking, which burns about 100 calories per mile, is as effective as running in reducing the risk of heart attack and stroke. It's even better than swimming because walking is a weight-bearing exercise, so it increases bone density, which helps prevent osteoporosis. Besides, walking is the simplest, most accessible form of exercise, and you can do it wherever you are, for the rest of your life. Remember that physical activity lowers homocysteine levels in the blood, so the more consistent you are with exercise, the more health benefits you'll receive.

Organized exercise is a good way to have company while you're sweating. Joining a gym that offers group classes, from yoga to stretching to spinning, provides a sense of community for some exercisers. If you're not in a big city, check out the local YMCA, churches, community centers, and schools— a lot of times they offer classes for which you pay one day at a time. Ask in a local sports shop where the swimming pools in town are; often you can start a swimming program by taking lessons. A personal trainer, though more expensive, can put you on a program that includes both strength and cardiovascular training. He or she may even come to your house.

Activities and Calories Burned Per Hour

Ballroom dancing	330
Bedmaking	234
Bicycling (five and a half miles per hour)	210
Bowling	264

Bricklaying	240
Carpentry	408
Desk work	132
Driving a car	168
Farm work in a field	438
Gardening	220
Golf	300
Handball and squash	612
Horseback riding (trot)	480
Ironing (standing up)	252
Lawn mowing (hand mower)	462
Preparing a meal	198
Roller skating	350
Running (ten miles per hour)	900
Scrubbing floors	216
Sitting and eating	84
Sitting in a chair reading	72
Skiing	594
Sleeping	60
Standing up	138
Sweeping the floor	102
Swimming (leisurely)	300
Tennis	420
Volleyball	350
Walking slowly (two and a half miles per hour)	216

Movers and Shakers: How to Keep Exercising

The second, crucial step in creating an exercise program is figuring out a way to keep doing it. Avoid the barriers that stop
you from exercising. Watching a lot of TV is a deterrent to
exercise, so don't turn it on. If you prefer exercising outdoors,
make sure you have an indoor alternative. If you like to

mountain bike but don't know where the trails are, go to the bike store and ask for trail maps or organized rides. Confidence in your ability to exercise will keep you motivated, which is why you're more likely to stick with a moderate-intensity activity than a high-intensity one.

There are certain proven methods of keeping exercise interesting. Setting a goal is one. Listening to music while you exercise is another. Keeping a written record of what you do will enable you to add up the calories you've burned (remember the 1,000 calories per week guideline for health benefits; 3,500 calories burned equals a pound of fat) and have a sense of achievement. Even buying exercise clothes and shoes you like will help get you out the door.

The human body is an amazing piece of machinery. Your body will respond to whatever you do by getting better at it. If you don't exercise at all right now, and want to start, it will take only about ten weeks of thirty minutes of accumulated exercise each day to achieve moderate fitness. That's not bad for decreasing your chances of disease and death.

Strength in Numbers: The Importance of Strength Training

So far, we've been talking about aerobic exercise—gardening, swimming, running, walking, cycling, all the forms of exercise that make you breathe hard and sweat. But resistance or strength training is important, too. By stressing the muscles when you're lifting weights or pushing against something or even using your own body weight, like leg lifts or push-ups, you're providing a different type of benefit from the cardiovascular training described as moderate and vigorous. Strength training builds lean muscle tissue and strengthens bones. You want to have as much lean muscle tissue as possible because it burns more calories at rest. A pound of muscle needs 20 calories per day to exist; a pound of fat needs only 2 calories. So the more muscle in your body, the more calories you will burn just sitting there.

Strength training has long-term health benefits as well. It may also reduce the risk of heart disease, non–insulin dependent diabetes, and certain types of cancer. In addition, it helps prevent osteoporosis by strengthening bones.

Your functional health is improved, too. When the muscles are strong, they take on the workload, not your joints. So when you are bending over to lift a heavy bag, walking up stairs, getting in and out of cars, these activities will place stress on the muscles, where it belongs, instead of on the joints and ligaments. Muscular fitness may be helpful in preventing upper and lower back pain. It also is important for the normal functioning of hormones and the metabolism of sugars, fatty acids, and amino acids. Having strong muscles gives you better balance, coordination, and agility that may help prevent falls when you're older.

It doesn't take a lot of work to increase your strength. The American College of Sports Medicine recommends one set of eight to ten exercises that condition all the major muscle groups, two or three days a week to prevent loss of muscle mass. When doing the exercises, eight to twelve repetitions of each is fine. The American College of Sports Medicine also suggests flexibility training—stretching major muscle groups—two or three days a week.

The Skinny on Fat: Why We're Obese

"As a nation, we've gone to pot-belly," wrote a reporter in the *Washington Post*. It's true. Over half of Americans are considered overweight or obese according to the 1998 guidelines of the National Heart, Lung, and Blood Institute. That means 97 million people. Over 3 million women weigh at least one hundred pounds over their ideal body weight.

It's a scary thought, especially when considering the consequences. The experts agree that obesity is associated with premature death. Next to smoking, inactivity and obesity are the second leading cause of preventable death. Obesity has been linked to heart disease, high blood pressure, diabetes, respiratory disease, arthritis, cancer, and gout. If we know the consequences, why do we as a nation continue to gain weight?

I've already explained why the low-fat diet doesn't work. Although it seems as if we've been eating less fat since the mid-1960s—we now eat 33 to 34 percent fat and we used to eat 40 percent—we're actually eating more fat. I'll tell you why. Because of our fat phobia, we've increased the actual number of total calories we consume. Most of them are in the form of refined carbohydrates. So even though we're consuming a smaller percentage of total calories in the form of fat, we're actually eating more fat because it's a percentage of a larger number. Our relative fat intake has gone down, but our total fat consumption, along with total calories, is up.

The bigger problem is that we are consuming so many carbohydrate calories—especially in the form of white flour and sugar products, as well as soft drinks. All carbohydrates turn to sugar or glucose in the body, and glucose is what the muscles and brain need the most. However, excess glucose is eas-

ily stored as fat. Unless you're burning off all those extra carbohydrate calories through exercise, they are stored as fat. It's
no coincidence that our relative carbohydrate consumption
is way up, and so is our weight.

The combination of greatly increased carbohydrate consumption, a higher total fat intake, and inactivity has made
the United States a country of very obese people. Physical
activity has declined in proportion to our growing waists.
We're using fewer calories than our ancestors—certainly far
fewer than our hunter-gatherer friends—and we're not com-
pensating for that difference with more exercise.

The Cat in the Hat Is Fat: Childhood and Adolescent Obesity

We're starting young. It is estimated that one in every five
children in this country is obese. The number of overweight
children has increased by almost 50 percent during the past
two decades, and the number of "extremely" overweight children has nearly doubled. Obesity is the number one nutritional disease of kids in this country. It's not hard to see why.
Children are less active than ever. They are playing video
games and sitting in front of computers. Participation in
physical education is down, time spent watching TV is up.
Only a third of children and teens eat the recommended
amounts of fruit, grain, meat, dairy, and vegetables.

This is disastrous for our children. There is a risk of eating
disorders, discrimination, negative self-image, depression,
and weight preoccupation, as well as increased risk of sleep
apnea, diabetes, and orthopedic complications. What's worse,
these children will most likely grow up to be obese adults,

developing severe conditions like elevated homocysteine levels, low HDL, high triglycerides, high blood pressure, changes in glucose and insulin sensitivity that predispose them to diabetes, gout, gallbladder disease, respiratory disease, cancer, arthritis, osteoporosis, and especially heart disease.

We must act as positive role models for our children. If we eat a healthy diet and are physically active, chances are our children will follow our example. Prevention is the best way to reduce obesity, and regular exercise will help that effort.

Getting Fit and Staying That Way

- Try to get thirty minutes of accumulated physical activity every day. The idea is to burn an extra 150 calories by combining any of the following: brisk walking, yard work, running, stair climbing, in-line skating, bicycling, dancing, swimming, bowling, playing tennis or volleyball, actively playing with children, jumping rope, or doing anything else that gets your heart rate up.

- Strength train two times per week, ideally. If you don't want to go to a gym, push-ups are the best exercise that you can do anywhere. Carrying heavy bags, standing then squatting, lifting a bar, doing dumbbell curls with water bottles, doing sit-ups, lifting heavy baskets in the garden, and doing leg lifts all count.

- It's important to stretch the major muscle groups every other day at least. It's best to stretch after your muscles are warmed up, not first thing in the morning while lying in bed.

- Try yoga.

- Set a goal for yourself: walking or running a five-kilometer race in the next four months; swimming thirty laps; participating in a walk-a-thon; cycling around your outdoor park; kayaking across a pond; hiking up a small mountain. Then keep a record of your daily training that is getting you to your goal.

- Exercise with a friend.

- If you go to the gym, take music with you.

- Read while walking on the treadmill.

- Commit to always taking the stairs instead of an elevator.

- Exercise first thing in the morning to get the day off to a good start.

- Ask the bike shop to put a more comfortable seat on your bike so you'll ride it more often.

- Find out about organized bike trips from your local sports shop.

- Call the Sierra Club in your state to learn about hiking trails.

- Buy new, supportive exercise shoes that you like.

- Wear exercise clothes that don't make you feel fat.

- Focus on being healthy, not thin.

8

Aging, Antioxidants, and Heart Disease

The Free Radical Theory and Thioretinaco Ozonide

The Heart Revolution describes how to prevent arteriosclerosis, heart disease, and heart attack, conditions that are strongly related to aging. Preventing these diseases will add healthy years to your life. But in doing so, is the process of aging itself somehow additionally slowed, halted, or reversed? Scientific understanding of the nature of aging is still fragmentary and incomplete. But insights about homocysteine's role in the body have recently culminated in a new theory, based on decades of scientific investigation, that explains how metabolism of homocysteine lies at the heart of the aging process.

The first theories of aging that promoted the idea of "wear and tear" of body tissues and organs were descriptive but too vague to be helpful. In the late 1930s experiments showed that deprivation of food calories significantly lengthens the life span of animals. A closely related discovery is that the ability of cells and tissues to use food energy by reaction with oxygen gradually declines with age. This "burning" of the hydrogen atoms of food with the oxygen of inhaled air, also known as cellular respiration, is the way living cells obtain chemical energy that is needed to fuel the basic processes of life itself. These early observations suggest that somehow the metabolism of calories from food by the oxygen of inhaled air is involved with the aging process.

We now recognize these observations as part of the free radical theory of aging. Introduced in the 1950s by Denham Harman as the radiochemical theory, "wear and tear" was described on a biochemical level as the declining ability of aging tissues to use oxygen and food. The theory states that the accumulation of oxygen radical compounds causes the aging of tissues and cells. Oxygen radicals are created when oxygen is used incompletely during cellular respiration. These highly reactive substances are capable of altering the chemical structure of many important biochemical constituents of the body. They react with unsaturated fats and cholesterol to produce cholesterol oxides that damage cell membranes. They make proteins less functional. And they break chromosomes and genes in DNA. The accumulation of excess free radical oxygen compounds is known as oxidative stress. Aging, then, can be defined as the many changes in cells, tissues, and organs that are the cumulative effect of damage by free radical oxygen compounds, or oxidative stress.

Before I move on to what can be done to prevent free radical damage, I want to explain how homocysteine is involved. In 1994 I introduced a closely related theory of aging that involves thioretinaco ozonide, a compound made of homocysteine, vitamin A, vitamin B12, and ozone. According to this theory, cells need thioretinaco ozonide to facilitate the process of cellular respiration. The theory states that during aging, thioretinaco ozonide is gradually lost from the membranes of cells, impairing their ability to convert free radical oxygen compounds to water. As a consequence, free radicals build up in cells and tissues, causing aging. The ability of cells to prevent accumulation of homocysteine also declines because of this loss of thioretinaco ozonide from cell membranes. Thioretinaco ozonide prevents formation of homocysteine from methionine in young cells by converting methionine to adenosyl methionine, a substance that is gradually lost from cells during aging. So not only is thioretinaco ozonide needed to prevent the accumulation of free radicals, it also keeps homocysteine low.

In addition, homocysteine inhibits the ability of thioretinaco ozonide to dispose of oxygen radicals by converting the substance to thioco, which has no effect on free radicals but instead promotes cellular growth. As you recall, the growth of muscle cells in artery walls produces arteriosclerotic plaques, leading to heart disease. The loss of thioretinaco ozonide from cell membranes during aging is closely regulated by many controlling factors inherited during millions of years of evolution. The nature of this regulation is not completely understood by medical scientists.

If thioretinaco ozonide is helping to keep our cells young, we want to do everything possible to nurture that compound, and a high level of homocysteine does the opposite. So in addition to causing damage to arteries, homocysteine is a major player in the aging process. One thing we can do to make as much thioretinaco ozonide as possible is to make sure we get enough of vitamins A and B12. We already have enough homocysteine.

As we age and lose our ability to absorb vitamin B6, folic acid, and vitamin B12, blood homocysteine levels rise, counteracting the ability of aging tissues to retain thioretinaco ozonide. By providing enough of these vitamins, the Heart Revolution diet facilitates the retention of thioretinaco ozonide in tissues, helping to delay the process of aging, as well as preventing arteriosclerosis and heart disease.

The Scavenger Hunt: Antioxidants and Aging

The plan for living longer is to decrease the amount of free radicals and increase the thioretinaco ozonide in cells. Since we are surrounded by an atmosphere containing the gas that creates the free radicals—oxygen—there must be a very potent chemical control system that keeps these destructive compounds at a low level. Luckily, there is. First of all, thioretinaco ozonide converts free radicals into water, creating the chemical energy that is used by cells. Secondly, our food contains antioxidant compounds—substances that neutralize free radicals, converting them to harmless by-products. Finally, our cells also contain several powerful enzymes (catalase, superoxide dismutase, glutathione peroxidase) that break down free radicals.

The best defense we have against free radicals is right in our cells—a substance called glutathione is the most potent antioxidant there is. Glutathione is made from three amino acids—glutamic acid, cysteine, and glycine—and is in every cell of the body. It can react with free radicals to form oxidized glutathione, which is a harmless compound that is converted back into glutathione within cells. Because of these reactions with free radicals, the balance between the amounts of glutathione and oxidized glutathione within cells is a measure of oxidative stress. Some nutritionists recommend glutathione supplements to help ensure against free radical buildup. While glutathione taken as a supplement is very safe, it is largely broken down into its constituent amino acids during digestion. For this reason, supplements have little effect on increasing the amount of glutathione within cells.

Our bodies also produce other compounds that help to eliminate free radicals—glucose, uric acid, bilirubin, and xanthine. Some experts believe that our bodies naturally build up these compounds during diseases like diabetes, gout, and liver disease to fight against the oxidative stress of free radicals within our cells.

Several of the vitamins in foods are themselves antioxidants. The most important ones are vitamins C, E, and A. As pointed out in Chapter Three, vitamin C is in many foods, especially fruits and leafy vegetables. Vitamin C acts with glutathione and thioretinaco ozonide inside cells to convert free radical oxygen into water, preventing damage to cells.

During metabolism, homocysteine, together with oxygen, is turned into sulfate with the help of vitamin C. If there isn't enough vitamin C, the reaction doesn't occur, homocysteine builds up, and sulfate is not formed from homocysteine. Sulfate is a mineral that is needed to help make connective tissues during normal growth. Excess sulfate is excreted in the urine.

When homocysteine builds up because of a lack of vitamin C, blood vessels start to disintegrate, blood platelets don't work properly, and the small blood vessels in the gums and skin start to hemorrhage. This is what we usually think of as a vitamin C deficiency—bleeding gums and bleeding in the skin.

In experimental animals with a vitamin C deficiency, a thin layer of fat is deposited in the lining of the aorta, the major artery of the body. However, arteriosclerotic plaques are not produced, and when vitamin C is restored, the fats from the aorta disappear and no plaques remain. Vitamin C is also needed for normal metabolism of homocysteine and helps to prevent accumulation of oxygen free radicals in cells and tissues. For these reasons, vitamin C helps to prevent homocysteine buildup in arteriosclerosis and retard the aging process. Vitamin C prevents deposition of fats in the aorta probably by decreasing the reaction of homocysteine with LDL, thereby decreasing formation of LDL homocysteine aggregates. These experiments suggest that vitamin C deficiency by itself doesn't cause arteriosclerosis.

Vitamin E is another important antioxidant. Vitamin E therapy was controversial for years, but recently it has been proven to lower the risk of heart attack by as much as 50 percent. Vitamin E, like other antioxidants, helps to delay arteriosclerosis by preventing the reaction of LDL with oxygen free radicals in early plaques. In this regard, vitamin E counteracts the effects of homocysteine in creating free radicals, preventing oxidant stress and decreasing the growth of arteriosclerotic plaques.

Missing Links: Other Antioxidants and Homocysteine

Essential oils from foods derived from plants and animals work as antioxidants, too. Because of their ability to react with free radicals, these unsaturated oils help to decrease oxidant stress and prevent damage to cells. Essential oils, like vitamin E, retard the formation of arteriosclerotic plaques because of this antioxidant effect. In addition, tests on patients with arteriosclerosis show that omega–3 unsaturated oil obtained from fish lowers the level of blood homocysteine. This action also helps to reduce oxidative stress, slowing down the aging process and preventing the formation of plaques by homocysteine. The fish that contain the most omega–3 unsaturated oils are salmon, tuna, and mackerel.

Another important unsaturated fat is the omega–6 fat that is in corn, safflower, peanut, and other plant oils. It helps to lower homocysteine, cholesterol, and LDL, and so it, too, will help prevent plaques in arteries. However, too much omega–6 fat and too little omega–3 fat can upset the beneficial balance of these essential oils, leading to inflammation, which is part of arteriosclerosis, arthritis, and colitis (see Chapter Four). Canola oil and olive oil are better choices as sources of unsaturated fats because they contain favorable ratios of omega–6 to omega–3 oils.

Ubiquinone, or coenzyme Q10, is an important antioxidant for prevention and treatment of heart disease. It's made in our bodies but it can also be obtained from the dietary fats and oils of fish, meat, and nuts. Some people even take coenzyme Q10 as a supplement to counteract oxidative stress. All cells of the body require ubiquinone to make energy when food is burned with oxygen. During this process, ubiquinone works with thioretinaco ozonide to produce chemical energy by converting oxygen to water. In doing so, ubiquinone functions as a powerful antioxidant, preventing free radicals from forming. And that's exactly what we want since it slows down the aging process. Furthermore, ubiquinone helps to counteract the oxidative stress from too much homocysteine within cells.

Too much homocysteine and too little ubiquinone prevents the heart muscle cells from producing enough chemical energy from food and oxygen. This results in heart failure. Ubiquinone therapy has been successful in reversing some forms of heart failure in which the heart muscle has partially lost its power to contract.

One of the big problems of the cholesterol-lowering statin drugs is that they inhibit cells from making ubiquinone normally. You should not ignore this important side effect when deciding whether to take these drugs. If you must take statin drugs, you should consider taking ubiquinone supplements, too.

Retinoids are potent antioxidants related to vitamin A. They are commonly found in carrots, green leafy vegetables, tomatoes, sweet potatoes, and other vegetables. The important retinoids, beta-carotene and lycopene, obtained from carrots and tomatoes, act directly to counteract free radicals. In the body retinoids are converted to vitamin A, which is also known as retinol. Vitamin A is essential for vision, normal immunity, fetal development, and normal growth and function of cells. Vitamin A also acts with B12 and homocysteine to produce thioretinaco ozonide, which, as discussed, is the complex that produces energy for cells and prevents the buildup of free radicals.

Bioflavonoids are another group of antioxidants from citrus fruits and garlic, onions, and other vegetables. These phytochemicals of foods derived from plants help counteract the oxidant stress of free radicals. One of them, troxerutin, has been proven, along with B6, folic acid, and B12, to reduce homocysteine, cholesterol, LDL, and triglycerides in people with heart disease. Troxerutin is derived from extracts of orange peels and is commonly taken as a supplement in Europe to counteract arteriosclerosis and blood clots in veins.

Other bioflavonoids include quercetin from fruit peels and pycnogenol from pine bark, sometimes taken as supplements; catechin from tea; and the polyphenols of red wine. These are just a few of the different compounds that we know have a positive effect on our cells. It's best to get these phytochemical antioxidants in fresh whole vegetables and fruits that are a staple of the Heart Revolution diet. Thousands of other antioxidant compounds from plants are being studied to see how they can prevent arteriosclerosis and oxidant stress.

Antioxidants are one way we know to slow down the aging process. Some experts advise taking large doses of antioxidant supplements, such as vitamin C, vitamin E, ubiquinone, and phytochemicals. Taken as supplements, these antioxidants are effective. But if eaten in whole foods, you will get thousands of other antioxidants also needed to delay aging. Antioxidant supplements can also be risky, because they are not balanced with other compounds, as they are in foods. Remember what happened with beta-carotene? It was first touted as an antioxidant, but then it was shown to increase the risk of lung cancer in smokers. No matter how they are taken, antioxidants are not a cure for aging; nothing can delay aging indefinitely.

You'll notice that all the antioxidants I mention are found in real plants that grow in the ground, not in refined, highly processed foods in the supermarket. And for every one we know about, probably a thousand other undiscovered antioxidants exist in food. It's one more reason to eat real, whole foods instead of processed junk food.

All the antioxidant vitamins, oils, and phytochemicals of the diet help to limit damage to cells by free radicals. In this respect these antioxidants help to retard the aging process. Indeed, there are people eating antioxidant-rich diets in certain parts of the world, such as Abkasia in the Caucasus Mountains, who achieve extraordinary longevity. Eating an optimal diet, as outlined in Chapter Four, will supply enough of these antioxidants to promote longevity. Longevity is achieved when arteriosclerosis and other degenerative diseases are suppressed. But no amount of antioxidants will extend your life span indefinitely. Future research is needed to find ways to prevent loss of thioretinaco ozonide from cells, retarding the process of aging.

Precautionary Measures: Avoiding Free Radicals

A diet rich in antioxidants will help wipe out free radicals. But there are other things we can do to prevent them in the first place. Have you ever noticed that your friends who smoke look the oldest? Even if they don't have emphysema or lung cancer, their skin shows signs of aging before that of their peers. When tobacco burns at a high temperature during smoking, the result is a lungful of free radicals. These free radicals damage lung tissue and are carried throughout the body, where they speed up the aging of skin and other tissues. In addition, we know that heavy smokers have a shortened life span because of their increased risk of cancer, heart disease, and lung disease. By quitting, you will reduce the risk of these diseases by eliminating the carcinogens, carbon monoxide, and other toxic substances in cigarette smoke. You will also eliminate free radicals from this source, preventing their aging effect on skin and preserving a more youthful appearance.

As for the diet, in addition to eating foods full of antioxidants, it's smart to avoid foods that contain or cause free radicals. Food that has been preserved through irradiation is rich in free radicals. The way radiation works is to flood the food with free radical oxygen compounds, devouring the antioxidants. Remember that this process also inactivates B6 and folic acid. Heavily smoked or grilled foods should also be avoided because the intense heat and smoke generate free radicals, found in the charred portion of the food.

And as I've mentioned a dozen times before, any food that contains oxy-cholesterols should be avoided. Heating meats, eggs, poultry, or fish to high temperatures, such as frying them in hot oil, not only turns the cholesterol in the food into harmful oxy-cholesterol, but produces a flood of free radical oxygen compounds.

Going the Distance: Diet, Aging, and Longevity

The Mediterranean Diet

Until her death in 1997, the oldest known human being in the world was a 126-year-old woman from Arles in Provence,

France. Two factors help to explain her extraordinary life span. First of all, her relatives and ancestors had long lives. Heredity is very important in determining longevity. But this woman also ate the "Mediterranean diet" her entire life. This diet—fresh vegetables, fruits, seafood, olive oil, red wine, garlic, herbs, and fiber—seems to promote health and longevity. Not only is it full of foods that are natural sources of antioxidants, but this nutritious diet provides the vitamins, minerals, essential oils, fiber, and phytochemicals that promote longevity. Many experts respect the Mediterranean diet and consider it the most healthful way of eating. The Heart Revolution diet, as explained in Chapter Four, is very similar to the traditional Mediterranean diet.

The proof of this diet's benefits can be observed in various populations. The death rate from heart disease in the southern and central European countries adjacent to the Mediterranean Sea—Spain, France, Italy, Portugal, and Greece—is one-third to one-fourth that of other European countries such as Scotland, Ireland, the Czech Republic, Finland, and Hungary. Why the difference? The usual explanation focuses on the variation in saturated fat content between the two diets, particularly when it comes to saturated fat from animals and dairy food. But northern Europeans eat more flour, sugar, and refined foods that cause a B vitamin deficiency. The Mediterranean diet supplies more B6 and folic acid that protect against heart disease by keeping homocysteine levels low. Southern Europeans, like the people in France, Greece, and Italy, also eat a lot of fat from olive oil and the monounsaturated oil and the omega–3 unsaturated fats in the olive oil are actually protecting them from disease.

France, of course, is the biggest wrench in the traditional

cholesterol argument because the French have a very high intake of saturated fats and cholesterol from meats and relatively high levels of blood cholesterol. Yet their incidence of heart disease is low—leading to the so-called French paradox.

The typical explanation of the French paradox is that since the French drink so much red wine, it must be the beneficial phytochemical antioxidants that prevent heart disease. This is true, but there's more to the story. Homocysteine explains the French paradox. In many parts of France, liver and other organ meats are very popular staples of the diet. Liver is the single best source there is of vitamin B6, folic acid, and vitamin B12. By eating pâté de foie gras, liver, and sweetbreads, the French consume large amounts of these three vitamins, and so prevent blood homocysteine levels from rising.

Of course, the other components of the traditional French diet—fresh vegetables and fruits, seafood, olive oil, red wine, garlic, and herbs—also contribute to prevention of heart disease by counteracting the damaging effects of homocysteine on arteries. All these foods not only contain phytochemical antioxidants, but they are also good sources of B6 and folic acid, so homocysteine levels are reduced even further.

Overall the French diet and the Mediterranean diet are good precursors to the Heart Revolution diet. The only significant difference between them and the diet I'm advocating is in the use of grains. The French baguette leaps to mind when most of us think of France. When we think of Italy, it's pasta. If the bread and pasta of these countries are made from freshly ground whole wheat, these foods are moderately good sources of vitamin B6 and folic acid. But a lot of times they're made from highly refined white flour that is depleted of these vitamins. European flours don't always have the same amount of preservatives and additives as the American versions do, but they're still depleted. In Europe, it's always better, as it is here, to opt for the multigrain breads, called *pane integrale* in Italy, and *pain complet* in France.

I'm not saying that we should eliminate these foods completely. Pasta is one of life's greatest pleasures. But I would like to strike a compromise. I suggest you eat only breads and pastas made from freshly ground whole grains. And they should be eaten not every day, but once in a while, since they may contribute to obesity when eaten in excess. In this way, the best parts of the French, Mediterranean, and Heart Revolution diets can be combined without too much sacrifice.

I hope that the Mediterranean countries can maintain their reliance on their high-quality traditional diets. If people living in these countries can resist the recent trend toward fast foods and refined processed foods, an increased risk of heart disease can be avoided in the future.

Asian countries, including Japan, China, Indonesia, and Thailand, also have a very low rate of coronary heart disease, and Japan leads the world in life expectancy. The traditional Asian diet is based on fresh vegetables and fruits, rice and other grains, and seafood. Their consumption of meat and dairy products is strictly limited. The advantage of this diet is that, first of all, they don't eat much methionine, which is turned into homocysteine in the body. They also eat an abundance of fresh vegetables and fruits, meaning they get enough B6 and folic acid to keep homocysteine levels low.

But the Asian diet is changing. As these countries become more Westernized, so have their diets. Japanese children are growing taller because they are eating more meat and dairy food, and the affluent adults in Japan have an increased rate of heart disease. If they continue to introduce more and more refined carbohydrates, the probability of disease will go in the direction of the United States and other high-risk populations—up.

Upping the Ante: The Effects of Minerals and Phytochemicals on Homocysteine

So now we know a few things. Our homocysteine levels increase as we age. The free radical scavenger thioretinaco ozonide decreases as we get older. According to the thioretinaco ozonide theory, susceptibility to arteriosclerosis and cancer increases as we age because of these two conditions. The loss of thioretinaco ozonide from cells makes them more likely to be transformed into malignant cells by chemical carcinogens, radiation, viruses, inflammation, and hormones. These carcinogens further reduce the level of thioretinaco ozonide in target cells; these cells are most affected by carcinogens and give rise to cancer cells. The result is altered cellular respiration and increased homocysteine production, causing the abnormal growth of cancer cells. In people who don't get enough B vitamins in their diet, the loss of thioretinaco ozonide from the cells of artery walls makes them more susceptible to arteriosclerosis by increased homocysteine levels. Either way, it's a bad combination.

Even though we don't presently have a way to restore thioretinaco ozonide to aging tissues, we can prevent homocysteine from building up, solving part of the problem. The degenerative diseases that result from too much homocysteine can be avoided, leaving the valuable thioretinaco ozonide alone to do its job. This strategy will help us live longer.

If heart disease alone were eliminated, overall life expectancy in America would increase. The following experiment proves this point. A small group of men with high blood cholesterol and coronary heart disease were given a combination of vitamin B6, folic acid, vitamin B12, riboflavin, troxerutin, and choline. Remember that troxerutin is an antioxidant and choline helps to convert homocysteine back to methionine. Over a period of only three weeks, this simple treatment produced a decline of blood homocysteine, cholesterol, triglycerides, and LDL by almost one-third. What this suggests is that a vitamin and antioxidant cocktail can stave off heart disease, therefore increasing longevity. These nutrients are supplied in the correct balance by the Heart Revolution diet.

I bring up this experiment to show that there are other elements, in addition to the B vitamins, that help control homocysteine. Their impact may not be as dramatic as B6, B12, and folic acid, but they are certainly important. This is another reason that it's preferable to get vitamins from food and not supplements, since all the other elements of the food may be helping to lower homocysteine and fight disease, too.

Earlier in this chapter I talked about the beneficial effects of phytochemicals like troxerutin on vascular disease because of their antioxidant properties. In this experiment troxerutin helped the B vitamins and other compounds to lower blood homocysteine and LDL levels. Riboflavin is a B vitamin that helps to produce chemical energy within cells. It is also essential since it converts folic acid into a form capable of turning homocysteine back into methionine, as shown in this experiment.

Two other substances found in food, betaine and choline, are capable of converting homocysteine back to methionine in our bodies. Choline is a part of lecithin, an emulsifying agent found in many foods including beans, meat, egg yolk, wheat germ, and yeast. The brain needs choline to function properly; choline also helps nerves and cell membranes to form normally. Betaine is found in a variety of foods, especially in beets. In the liver, choline and betaine convert homocysteine to methionine by a separate enzymatic pathway. These substances help to lower blood homocysteine in patients with heart disease independently of vitamin B6, folic acid, and vitamin B12.

Again, this is why getting our vitamins from food is preferable to taking supplements alone. Many other constituents in food can help to fight disease, and yet we know about only a small percentage of them. Take, for example, minerals. The food we eat contains many minerals, and some are being tested for their preventive properties.

Minerals like iron, copper, magnesium, zinc, cobalt, and selenium contribute to lowering free radicals in the body and slowing the aging process. Instead of taking these minerals in supplements, you can get them from whole grains and fresh vegetables. You may know that iron is needed to make the hemoglobin pigments of red blood cells, the myoglobin of muscle, and the enzymes that carry oxygen during cellular respiration. Not only does iron speed up reactions with oxygen, it also speeds the reaction of LDL with free radicals, producing oxy-cholesterols in arteriosclerotic plaques. Furthermore, homocysteine increases the ability of iron to speed the reaction of free radicals with LDL. Recent studies have suggested that too much iron may increase the risk of heart disease. For this reason, older men and postmenopausal women should avoid taking iron supplements unless they are anemic.

Copper is an essential mineral, but too much copper is

unhealthy. Like iron, it produces free radicals and also increases the amount of oxy-cholesterols from LDL in plaques. LDL, as you remember, carries homocysteine to the artery walls, so it can increase the risk of heart disease. But too little copper leads to overproduction of cholesterol and LDL, as well as weakness of artery walls. A simple blood test can tell you if you have the right amount.

Magnesium activates the coenzymes and enzymes that are needed to excrete homocysteine from the body. Another important mineral, cobalt, is an essential part of vitamin B12 that converts homocysteine back to methionine. It is also the element of thioretinaco ozonide that converts free radical oxygen to water and chemical energy. Selenium is a component of the enzyme glutathione peroxidase that inactivates many different free radical substances in the body. Zinc enables the enzymes of cellular respiration to function and helps to prevent excessive formation of free radicals. Manganese is a component of the enzyme superoxide dismutase that breaks down oxygen free radicals.

Several minerals, especially cobalt, manganese, and selenium, can directly reduce free radical buildup, preventing heart disease and certain effects of aging. But minerals, like vitamins, are depleted from processed grains, as explained in Chapter Three. Therefore we need to add them back to our diets. Drinking hard water, even though it has a mineral taste, is one such way—but this only works in areas where tap water is rich in dissolved minerals.

Overall, our bodies need a delicate balance of vitamins, antioxidants, phytochemicals, antioxidant oils, fiber, choline, and minerals. If you are eating depleted food and popping a few supplements, you may be missing out on the proper balance of the other nutrients in food. Most people worry that they eat too much, but, really, the question is: Are you eating enough of the right foods?

Beat the Clock: Living Longer and Healthier

As a culture, we are obsessed with youth. But as we get older and accept the inevitable loss of youth, we cling tenaciously to the idea of just plain living longer. We try pills, potions, even plastic surgery to either extend our lives or delude ourselves into thinking we have.

For decades some people have been taking various hormones to postpone aging, but none of these treatments has been proven to extend life span or to offer eternal youth. A great example is the recent interest in dehydroepiandrosterone (DHEA), a hormone that declines with age. Some people are taking DHEA supplements, which can be bought in health food stores. But many doctors warn against taking DHEA because of potential harmful side effects. Another example is human growth hormone (hGH). Some people pay thousands of dollars a month to be injected by hGH in a doctor's office. The logic is that DHEA and hGH production, as well as other hormones such as melatonin, testosterone in men, and estrogen in women, declines with age. By replenishing them, people hope they will reverse the aging process. Although these hormones indeed decrease as we age, this doesn't explain *why* we age. The decrease in these hormones is a *symptom* of aging. But we can't stop aging by taking a few synthetic versions of our natural hormones. One theory, the neuroendocrine theory, hypothesized that aging is the result of changes in the secretion of hormones. But these decreases are the *consequence* of aging, not the cause. Ultimately this theory doesn't hold because it doesn't explain the change in food metabolism or accumulation of free radical compounds with age.

The free radical theory is now widely accepted as the cause of aging. In my view, the key lies in thioretinaco ozonide. If ways can be found to stabilize thioretinaco ozonide, perhaps its loss from cells can be prevented. Preserving thiroteinaco ozonide will keep free radical production at a low level, retarding the aging process. This may be the only way to extend the human life span.

For now the one thing we know we can do to live longer is to put the brakes on the diseases that shorten our lives. It is possible to prevent heart disease, cancer, diabetes, senile dementia, arthritis, and diseases of the liver, kidney, and lungs. In fact a 1998 study found that blood homocysteine is elevated in victims of Alzheimer's disease because of inadequate B vitamins. Certainly in this book I've shown you how easy it is to prevent heart disease by eating enough B6, folic acid, B12, and other nutrients to keep homocysteine levels low.

Many studies have shown that eating more fruits and vegetables, fiber, and other nutrients reduces the risk of heart disease, cancer, hypertension, and other degenerative diseases. The Heart Revolution diet will do just that. And by controlling free radicals, this diet counteracts the oxidative stress induced by increased levels of homocysteine in the blood, cells, and tissues.

I can't promise that your wrinkles will go away, your gray hair will disappear, and your energy will be the same today as it was when you were twenty. But the Heart Revolution can slow down the aging process—considerably—and prevent disease—definitely. You'll live longer, be healthier, and age more gracefully.

9

The Future of the Revolution

A New Outlook

By reading this book, you now have a better understanding of what causes heart disease. The homocysteine approach to disease—and aging—requires a new way of looking at what goes on in our bodies, and especially our arteries. This idea forces us to reexamine the cholesterol hypothesis as myth. Now we know that the cholesterol and fats in arteriosclerotic plaques are only a symptom of heart disease, not the cause. Homocysteine, not cholesterol, is the culprit.

This is a revolutionary way of looking at heart disease. It's the opposite of what the cholesterol camp would have us believe. Heart disease is caused not by an *excess*—overcon-sumption of fats and cholesterol—but by a nutritional *defi-ciency*—lack of vitamins B6, folic acid, and B12. To prevent the disease, the emphasis needs to be on supplying adequate nutrients in our food, not on limiting fat and cholesterol.

It's time to revise our thinking. The idea that eating too much fat and cholesterol raises the LDL and blood choles-terol is outmoded. We have seen that the homocysteine approach explains changes in LDL and HDL as symptoms and not causes of heart disease. Fats and cholesterol are not the demons in our food supply. But, ironically, our fear of them has made us eat more of the true villains—refined flour, sugar, and other processed foods. The low-fat, low-cholesterol diet is propelling us to eat more of the very foods that cause our B vitamin deficiencies. No wonder the United States is filled with obese, diabetic, hypertensive people, and heart disease is the number one killer among men and women. Many people in this country are in a state of nutritional disaster.

Until recently homocysteine has been the underdog of the research world. Thankfully in the 1990s homocysteine is being studied more extensively than it was in the past three decades. The conclusion? It seems that homocysteine is involved in every aspect of heart disease: the overgrowth of muscle cells that hardens the arteries; fibrosis and calcifica-tion of plaques; deposition of cholesterol and fats in plaques; and, finally, blockage of the arteries by blood clots. Homocysteine is the missing link that explains all the known risk factors of heart disease: aging, genetic predisposition, hormonal factors, smoking, toxins, exercise, drugs, and, of course, diet. Homocysteine is the answer research has been looking for.

Homocysteine and the Brain

Researchers from around the world are now investigating homocysteine to see what role it may play in other diseases. Some of the most exciting studies have looked at the way homocysteine affects the brain, specifically the aging brain. In the next section, I'll briefly summarize some of the intriguing findings and what is on the horizon as we learn more about the extensive part homocysteine may take in diseases ranging from Alzheimer's to arthritis.

Alzheimer's Disease and Homocysteine

One of the most devastating, feared, and common diseases of the brain is Alzheimer's disease. In this condition of dementia, the ability of the brain to remember recent events begins to decline, and gradually other mental capacities are lost over a period of months or years. The final result of this disease is an elderly person who is unable to recognize close family members, unable to care for himself, and unable to carry out even the simplest tasks.

Although Alzheimer's disease usually occurs in the elderly, generally in the seventh and later decades, it may strike at an earlier age, particularly when there is a family history of early onset of the disease. The underlying cause of Alzheimer's is incompletely understood by medical scientists, but there are some factors that seem to predispose certain people, including a family history, high fat consumption, and a variation of a lipoprotein found in the blood (ApoE4). Additionally, the results of an Oxford University study published in 1998 showed that homocysteine may factor in as well. In this study, elevated blood homocysteine, along with dietary deficiencies of folic acid and vitamin B12, were implicated as important risk factors for Alzheimer's disease. This new information suggests that if we control our homocysteine levels by eating the Heart Revolution diet and taking dietary supplements we may be able to prevent this dreaded disease. It is certainly worth a try.

In support of these findings, other studies have also shown that many victims of Alzheimer's disease have a deficiency of vitamin B12. Unfortunately for patients, therapy with vitamin B12 is ineffective in reversing the brain damage. Other abnormal brain conditions in the elderly, including confusion and other types of dementia, were also found to be associated with low vitamin B12 levels in the blood. The good news is that some of these patients do respond to therapy with vitamin B12.

Vitamin Deficiencies and the Brain

Recent studies of brain function in general show clearly that high levels of blood homocysteine are associated with decreased mental ability—including fading memory, difficulty with language, and slowed perception. In studies, subjects with deficiencies of vitamin B6, folic acid, and vitamin B12 performed poorly in tests of certain mental functions compared with subjects without vitamin deficiencies. As explained earlier, these vitamin deficiencies increase the blood levels of homocysteine. This, in turn, impairs mental function by affecting the activity and survival of nerve cells in the brain.

An interesting example of homocysteine's relationship to

the brain goes back to the disease homocystinuria. If you remember from Chapter One, the original discovery of the disease homocystinuria resulted from examining homocysteine levels in the urine of children with mental retardation. There is more than one form of homocystinuria, each with a different underlying cause. In one type, the vast majority of children afflicted are mentally retarded. These children have not been helped with therapy to lower homocysteine levels. But in another type, caused by a deficiency of methylenetetrahydrofolate reductase, some of the afflicted children have mental symptoms closely resembling schizophrenia. In a few cases, these symptoms dramatically improved or disappeared with folic acid therapy.

In a recent study of patients with schizophrenia, about half were found to have distinctly elevated levels of blood homocysteine compared with normal subjects. Earlier studies had shown that many persons with schizophrenia metabolize methionine abnormally. As you recall, methionine is converted into homocysteine in the body. In experiments, when a large dose of methionine is injected or given by mouth, symptoms of schizophrenia are dramatically exacerbated. This occurs because the methionine immediately increases the homocysteine levels in the blood, although it is unclear precisely how homocysteine affects the brain. While these studies show a relation between homocysteine and schizophrenia, no effective therapy has yet been devised to treat or prevent the disease using diet or supplements. In some cases, the Heart Revolution diet may potentially help the condition by lowering homocysteine overall.

Deficiencies of vitamin B6, folic acid, and vitamin B12, particularly among older people, have been associated with a wide

range of mental disturbances and abnormalities including depression, irritability, confusion, and convulsions. Recent surveys have demonstrated a deficiency of folic acid in about one
third of patients with acute psychiatric disorders. Intriguingly,
therapy with folic acid (methyltetrahydrofolic acid) did improve their schizophrenic and depressive symptoms.

Deficiency of vitamin B12 in the elderly causes a variety
of neurological and psychiatric symptoms, including abnormal sensations, mental confusion, memory loss, unsteady
gait, weakness, and depression. Elevated levels of blood
homocysteine seem to play a role here, and therapy with vitamin B12 has been proven effective in treating elderly patients
with even borderline deficiencies.

Deficiency of vitamin B6 causes irritability, convulsions,
confusion, and depression in infants and adults. Drugs that
cause elevation of blood homocysteine levels by inhibiting
the body's ability to utilize vitamin B6, such as certain antibiotics, cause many of these mental symptoms as side effects,
and therapy with vitamin B6 improves these symptoms dramatically. Again, deficiency of vitamin B6 causes elevation of
blood homocysteine levels after meals, producing abnormal
brain function over a period of months or years.

Recent advances in understanding the function of the
brain have offered explanations of how homocysteine may
cause a wide variety of abnormalities of brain and nerve function. When animals are injected with large doses of homocysteine they go into convulsions, and some children with
homocystinuria suffer from convulsions as well. In the body,
homocysteine is converted into two related substances, homo-
cysteic acid and homocysteine sulfinic acid. Both substances
accelerate the transmission of neural signals and impulses.

Worse still, they oppose the action of certain inhibitory neurotransmitters, causing widespread abnormalities of brain and nerve function. One way in which homocysteine causes toxicity to the brain is to overstimulate membrane receptors (N-methyl-D-aspartate receptors), causing calcium to accumulate within nerve cells, antagonizing the action of nitric oxide, and increasing production of oxygen radicals. In plain language this means that the elevation of homocysteine—whether associated with deficiencies of B vitamins, drug therapy, Alzheimer's disease, or normal aging—contributes to damage of nerve tissues in our brains, nerves, and spinal cord.

Fibromyalgia and Chronic Fatigue Syndrome

A recently recognized syndrome, fibromyalgia, is actually a group of disorders characterized by muscle pain and stiffness, and a persistent, debilitating fatigue. A closely related condition known as chronic fatigue syndrome was recognized by the Centers for Disease Control in 1988. In both syndromes, patients complain of incapacitating fatigue lasting for more than six months, often along with fever or chills, sore throat, painful lymph nodes, muscle weakness, headaches, joint pain, neuropsychological disturbances, and sleep abnormalities. Fibromyalgia and chronic fatigue syndrome are closely related conditions, and no one yet knows the cause of either.

A 1997 study from Sweden found that subjects suffering from fibromyalgia and chronic fatigue had elevated homocysteine levels in their cerebrospinal fluid, the fluid which surrounds the brain. Most people in the study also had low or low normal levels of vitamin B12 in the cerebrospinal fluid, possibly accounting for the abnormal level of homocysteine. While these findings are intriguing, they have not yet led to an effective therapy for fibromyaligia or chronic fatigue syndrome.

Immunity and Infection

It probably comes as no news that vitamin deficiencies can lead to immune system problems and increased susceptibility to infection. How does this relate to homocysteine? Well, as you've already read in this book, elevated levels of homocysteine (frequently caused by vitamin deficiencies) can lead to plaque formation in the arteries. But in the past two decades, pathologists have also detected a variety of infectious organisms (including the herpes virus, chlamydia, and cytomegalovirus) in arterial arteriosclerotic plaques. For a variety of reasons, these infected plaques are sequestered from the cells and antibodies that would normally carry out the immune response. Thus, these organisms are able to grow unimpeded by the body's immune system. Many scientists believe that the growth of these agents within plaques can complicate the clogging of the arteries as arteriosclerosis becomes advanced. Of course, when the immune response is further suppressed by deficiencies of B and other vitamins, infectious agents can get into arteriosclerotic plaques and flourish.

Another area of research involves ulcers. Within the past two decades, our thinking about ulcers has changed. It used to be that ulcers were linked to diet, alcohol, smoking, and stress, and sufferers were urged to relax, take antacids, and stick to a bland diet. Recent studies have shown that in fact ulcers are most frequently caused by the bacteria *Helicobacter pylori*, which takes up residence in the lining of the stomach, causing inflammation and ulceration. How does homocysteine factor in? Recent studies have linked infection with *Helicobacter pylori* and peptic ulcer disease to increased susceptibility to coronary heart disease. As the lining of the stomach becomes inflamed and damaged, its ability to absorb both folic acid and vitamin B12 is sorely compromised—leading to, you guessed it, B vitamin deficiency and elevation of homocysteine. If you suspect you have an ulcer, it is important to have it promptly and properly treated to prevent nutrient deficiencies and subsequent elevation of homocysteine.

Autoimmune Diseases

Homocysteine may also play a role in autoimmune diseases, where the immune system reacts against and attacks the body's own tissues. A common form is rheumatoid arthritis, an autoimmune disease that causes pain, disability, and deformity in all joints of the body. Occurring rarely in childhood, the disease becomes increasingly common with age. Rheumatoid arthritis is associated with severe nutritional abnormalities, including low levels of vitamin B6. However, unfortunately for the millions of sufferers, therapy with vitamin B6 has no benefit in treating the disease. A 1997 study also found that patients with rheumatoid arthritis have elevated levels of homocysteine in the blood. Given this finding, it is hardly surprisingly that people with this disease frequently die from coronary heart disease or stroke. But at present it isn't clear whether nutritional or vitamin therapy to lower homocysteine levels will prevent rheumatoid arthritis or these vascular complications.

Lupus erythematosus is another autoimmune disease, one in which the immune system goes on the attack against a certain kind of DNA circulating in the blood. As with rheumatoid arthritis, many people suffering from lupus die from stroke, heart attack, and peripheral vascular disease. A 1996 study showed that the risk of vascular complications in lupus erythematosus is directly related to elevation of blood homocysteine levels. Scientists are presently studying whether therapy with vitamin B6, folic acid, and vitamin B12 will prevent vascular disease in patients suffering from lupus erythematosus.

The risk of autoimmune diseases like rheumatoid arthritis and lupus erythematosus rises steadily with age, even while immune response declines in most people. As explained in Chapter Eight, the level of homocysteine in the blood gradually rises with age. While it is not yet entirely clear, some studies suggest that there is a link between homocysteine levels and autoimmune response. It may be that homocysteine reacts with proteins, DNA, and other components of cells to alter their chemical properties. The immune system, sensing something new and different, kicks into gear to counter this challenge, not recognizing that it is attacking its own cellular material. Controlling homocysteine levels through the Heart Revolution diet may help to alleviate or prevent autoimmune diseases by preventing this inappropriate immune response.

Research both on brain and immune function has demonstrated the complex role that homocysteine plays in the body. While it is too early to suggest that Alzheimer's or autoimmune diseases can be prevented solely through lowering homocysteine levels, it certainly isn't a bad place to start. It is my hope that this book has inspired you to try the Heart Revolution diet to prevent heart disease and, if these promising studies bear fruit, to stave off many other diseases normally attributed to aging.

A Call to Action

Now that we know how heart disease is caused, we have insight into why this disease has been killing Americans in such dramatic numbers. As our food becomes more and more processed, we are consuming higher and higher amounts of refined carbohydrates such as white flour, white rice, and sugar, as well as chemically altered foods such as transfats, oxy-cholesterols, and irradiated products. What's missing from our diets is the food that our bodies are biologically equipped for—fish, meat, vegetables, fruits, whole grains, nuts, beans—the foods that contain B6, folic acid, B12, antioxidants, essential oils, minerals, fiber, and all the other nutrients that keep homocysteine levels low.

On an individual level, you can have your homocysteine checked to see how you're doing. Your doctor can send a simple blood sample to a commercial laboratory or a medical center to determine the level in your blood. A test that was introduced in 1998 makes homocysteine testing available in any hospital laboratory. Then, by following the Heart Revolution diet, you can protect yourself from a high homocysteine level and all its complications.

On a public health level, it's urgent that changes are made in our food supply to counteract the nutritional deficiencies that are causing the problems. Refined flour and sugar can be fortified; hydrogenated oils could be eliminated. The consequences of milling grains, sterilizing, and irradiating foods are the devastating losses of nutrients. These processes need to be corrected. Improving our methods of food production, processing, preservation, storage, distribution, and labeling is crucial to preventing vascular disease in this country. There should be a thorough review of industry practices and methods. Food scientists and the food industry must figure out a way to improve the nutritional value of our food.

Our consciousness has to change, too. The nutritional advice Americans hear every day is off base. The official government and health agencies are giving out confusing, contradictory, and inadequate messages. Have you ever heard a warning that refined foods are harmful to your health? I haven't. The dangers of highly processed foods and the depleted nature of white flour and sugar need to be communicated to the American public. People need to know how crucial it is that they consume fresh whole foods. What are we waiting for?

In epidemiological studies of thousands of people, deficiencies of the key vitamins—B6, folic acid, and B12—were proven to increase deaths from heart disease. So why hasn't anything been done about changing the RDA for B6? Or requiring adequate fortification of refined foods with B6, folic acid, and B12? Why does the Food Pyramid promote consumption of refined carbohydrates over beneficial fats that contain essential nutrients?

Unfortunately our food has become a political hot potato. With special interest councils and organizations created to promote certain food groups, the real measures that would help the population fight disease are debated, discussed, and often brushed aside. It's easier to go with the status quo than to change an entire country's mindset.

I disagree. There is an urgency to this matter. There are 500,000 people dying every year from heart disease, and millions more suffering with the disease and its related conditions. The reluctance of the Food and Nutrition Board of the National Research Council to amend its policies and add vital nutrients to refined and processed foods is unacceptable. The Dietary Guidelines, the Food Pyramid, and the RDA of B6 must change to reflect what we know about disease prevention. I believe the RDA for vitamin B6 should be increased to 3 milligrams per day for every adult. The RDA for folic acid of 400 micrograms per day needs to be fully supplied to the population by fortifying refined foods more adequately. This is a life-and-death situation. We are in a crisis, and action needs to be taken immediately.

Survival of the Fittest: Evolution and the Heart Revolution

If we don't take action, biology will do it for us. Already we can see that how we eat plays a part in natural selection. Heart disease, arteriosclerosis, cancer, and diabetes are limiting our survival. Those who can avoid these diseases live the longest. In certain cases of diabetes, high blood pressure, and coronary heart disease in young adults, the conditions prevent the weakest from reproducing.

Evolution plays a significant role in how our bodies metabolize food in the first place. We are not so different from our Paleolithic ancestors. We have inherited the same metabolic machinery from them that was a result of millions of years of evolution. Their diet—fish, meat, vegetables, fruits, seeds, and nuts—is our ideal diet. But, unfortunately, that's not how we eat. In recent history, say in the past 10,000 years, our diet has changed to include grains. Evolution doesn't work that fast. Our bodies are not well equipped to handle the foods that are grain-based. And certainly not the foods that have been created in the past hundred years, such as white flour and refined sugar. We haven't adapted to this diet, and that's where the trouble starts.

Knowing what we know, however, this awkward transition of waiting for our bodies to evolve doesn't have to kill us. We have the scientific means to study our diets. We know how crucial certain nutrients are to our health. And we have the information pathways to communicate this information to everyone. We can make the technological and nutritional changes so that our bodies and our food supply are in sync.

Although the individual dieting changes I'm suggesting may seem small and simple to accomplish—ordering a salad instead of french fries, eating multigrain rolls instead of white bread, eliminating partially hydrogenated oils—the collective consequences are tremendous. Your chance of getting heart disease, arteriosclerosis, and other vascular diseases will go down, but so will the risk of cancer, diabetes, and arthritis. The epidemic of obesity, hypertension, diabetes, and heart disease can be abated if enough of the population eats the Heart Revolution diet. We'll live longer, and enjoy better health while we're at it. All socioeconomic groups will benefit from better health, and as a result we'll see improvements in education and crime rates; there will be fewer people smoking, abusing alcohol, and taking drugs.

Revolutionary advances in medicine have had major impacts on societies in the past. Now we are in the unique position of knowing how to prevent heart disease and increase longevity. We just have to apply what we know, on an individual level, a national level, and an international level. Most important, the Heart Revolution can change not only how we live, but how future generations survive. Let the Heart Revolution be your opportunity for improving your own health and the health of your loved ones.

Appendix: Recipes

Heart Revolution Recipes

The recipes in this section will help you on the path to healthy eating. Unlike typical diet books, the focus here is on delicious foods that will leave you satisfied. The purpose is to make sure you're getting enough of the vitamins needed to prevent heart disease—B6, B12, and folic acid, as well as essential phytochemicals, fat-soluble vitamins, minerals, antioxidants, and essential oils. It is easy to follow this plan because it doesn't depend upon obscure ingredients only found in remote corners of big city stores, but on fresh, whole foods that are available just about everywhere.

Over the past thirty years, we've created and adapted recipes so that they provide the optimal nutrients for lowering homocysteine, while still tasting good. The following recipes are a few my family has enjoyed; they are for everyday living, as well as entertaining and special occasions. I guarantee that these foods will leave you—and your taste buds—fully satisfied.

Salads

Wheatberry Salad with Beets, Apricots, and Walnuts

½ pound dried apricots
½ cup apple cider
¼ cup fresh lemon juice
¼ cup fresh orange juice
1 tablespoon grated orange rind
½ teaspoon salt, plus more to taste
1 teaspoon freshly ground pepper
1 cup wheatberries, soaked in cold water overnight, then drained
4 cups chicken broth
6 medium beets, rinsed and scrubbed
8 shelled walnuts, lightly toasted, finely chopped
½ cup minced parsley leaves
2 tablespoons walnut oil

Combine the apricots and apple cider in a small bowl. Soak until plumped, about 1 hour. Drain, finely chop, and set aside.

In a separate bowl, whisk together the lemon juice, orange juice, and orange rind to make a vinaigrette. Season with some of the salt and pepper to taste. Set aside.

Combine the wheatberries and chicken broth in a saucepan. Bring to a boil, then reduce heat to medium-low and simmer until partially cooked, about 15 minutes. Drain. Add to the vinaigrette, toss, and set aside.

Combine the beets and 3 cups of cold water in a saucepan. Bring to a boil, reduce heat to medium, and simmer until tender, but not soft, about 20 minutes. Drain and rinse under cold water until cool. Peel and cut into ½-inch dice. Add to the salad, and toss. Add the apricots, walnuts, and parsley, and toss. Drizzle with walnut oil and toss again. Season with the remaining salt and pepper, or to taste. Serves 4.

Warm Quinoa Salad

¼ cup fresh lemon juice
1 tablespoon grated lemon rind
½ teaspoon salt, plus more to taste
1 teaspoon freshly ground pepper
1 tablespoon hazelnut oil
1 ripe pear, cored and cut into ¼-inch dice
1 apple, cored and cut into ¼-inch dice
¼ cup fresh lime juice
1 cup quinoa
1 bay leaf
3 sprigs fresh thyme
2 cups chicken or vegetable broth, preferably homemade
½ cup chopped cilantro leaves
¼ cup minced parsley leaves
Salt
Freshly ground pepper

To make a vinaigrette, combine lemon juice, lemon rind, salt, and pepper in a large bowl. Whisk in hazelnut oil. Set aside.

In a separate bowl, combine the pear, apple, and lime juice. Set aside.

Rinse the quinoa under cold running water in a strainer. Combine the quinoa, bay leaf, thyme, and broth in a small saucepan over high heat. Bring to a boil. Reduce the heat to medium-low, cover and simmer until tender and translucent, about 12–15 minutes. Remove and discard the bay leaf and thyme sprigs.

Add the warm quinoa to the vinaigrette. Add the pear and apple mixture and toss. Add the cilantro and parsley leaves and toss until combined. Season with salt and pepper to taste. Serves 4.

Greens and Brown Rice Salad

8 cups chopped arugula or watercress
¾ cup chopped, pitted oil-cured black olives
¾ teaspoon minced lemon rind
1 cup fresh lemon juice
2 ½ tablespoons olive oil
2 teaspoons salt, plus more to taste
Freshly ground pepper
3 cups cooked brown rice

In a large bowl, toss together the arugula or watercress, olives, lemon rind, lemon juice, and olive oil. Toss in the brown rice. Season with salt and pepper. Serves 6.

Hors-D'oeuvres

Roasted Nuts

1 pound nuts (almonds, pecans, Brazil nuts, hazelnuts, or walnuts)
2 tablespoons butter, softened
Salt
Freshly ground pepper (optional)

Preheat oven to 300 degrees F. Toss nuts with soft butter.

Roast for about 45 minutes, stirring every 10–15 minutes, until nuts turn brown. Serve warm or at room temperature. Remove from oven and toss with salt (pepper optional). Shake off excess salt and allow to cool. Serve at room temperature. Store in covered containers to insure freshness.

Chicken Liver Spread

1 tablespoon butter
1 large onion, preferably Vidalia, chopped fine
1 pound chicken livers
1 hard boiled egg
Salt
Freshly ground black pepper

Melt the butter in a fry pan over medium heat. Add the onion and cook until wilted, about 7 minutes.

Add chicken livers and cook until opaque. Remove from heat and add hard boiled egg. Place in the bowl of a food processor, and pulse until desired consistency is reached. Season to taste with salt and pepper.

Chill before serving on Wasa bread or endive leaves.

Guacamole

2 ripe avocados, peeled and pitted
2 teaspoons minced scallions
1 garlic clove
¼ teaspoon chili powder
Salt
Juice of 1 lemon
Optional ingredients: ½ cup chopped fresh cilantro, ¼ teaspoon red pepper flakes, ¼ cup chopped red onion, ¼ cup chopped tomato, ¼ chopped black olives

Rub a small bowl with the salt and a peeled garlic clove. Discard garlic. In the bowl mash avocados, chili powder, and lemon juice. Stir in chopped scallions. Optional ingredients may be added at this time. Cover tightly with plastic wrap and chill until serving time. Stir well before serving.

White Bean Spread

2 cups uncooked cannellini beans
2 sage leaves
½ teaspoon crushed red pepper flakes
2 teaspoons minced garlic
2 tablespoons olive oil
Fresh rosemary sprigs

Soak beans in cold water for an hour. Drain, place in a large stock pot with sage leaves, and add fresh water to cover by one inch. Bring to a boil over high heat, then reduce heat, cover, and simmer until soft, approximately one hour. They may need to cook up to 30 minutes more. Add additional water to cover as necessary. When the beans have cooked completely, drain and rinse with cold water.

Heat olive oil in a large sauté pan over medium heat. Add garlic, rosemary, and pepper and cook until garlic is golden brown. Add beans and cook over low heat for about 10 minutes, until beans are thoroughly coated and cooked through.

Remove rosemary sprigs. Place mixture in the bowl of a food processor or blender, and process for 30 seconds or until desired consistency is reached.

Chill until ready to use. Serve with Wasa bread.

Soups

Lentil Soup

6 cups chicken broth
1½ cups uncooked lentils, rinsed and picked over
1 cup uncooked brown rice
2 pounds tomatoes, peeled and chopped
3 carrots, peeled and diced
1 onion, finely chopped
1 celery stalk, chopped
3 garlic cloves, minced
½ teaspoon dried oregano

½ cup minced parsley
2 tablespoons red wine vinegar

Place all ingredients, except the parsley and vinegar, in a large stock pot. Bring to a boil over high heat. Reduce heat and simmer, stirring occasionally, until lentils are tender but not mushy, about 45 minutes.

Add parsley and vinegar just before serving. Serves 6–8.

Note: This recipe may be halved or doubled with very good results.

Cold Borscht

2 pounds beets, scrubbed
1 quart buttermilk
2 tablespoons lemon juice
1 small onion, chopped
Salt
A handful of chives, chopped

Steam beets until tender when pierced with fork, about 20 minutes. Under cold running water, peel beets, then chop into ½-inch cubes.

Place beets in the bowl of a food processor. Add 2 cups buttermilk and pulse 30 seconds or until beets are finely chopped. Add lemon juice and chopped onion and process again until smooth. Add remaining buttermilk and process again until all ingredients are incorporated. Season with salt to taste.

Chill until ready to serve. Garnish with chives. Serves 4–6.

Vegetable Soup with Beans

2 tablespoons olive oil
1 medium onion, chopped
2 cloves garlic, minced
½ teaspoon oregano
2 medium carrots, chopped
2 celery stalks, chopped
5 cups chicken stock

4 cups water

1 cup cooked chick peas (or red beans, kidney beans, or white
    beans), drained and rinsed

2 parsnips, peeled and chopped into ½-inch cubes (optional)

2 potatoes, peeled and chopped into ½-inch cubes (optional)

1 medium tomato, seeded and chopped

In a 4 quart stock pot, sauté onion, garlic, and oregano in olive oil until onion is wilted. Add the carrots and celery and sauté 5 minutes more.

Add chicken stock, water, and beans. Bring to a boil. Reduce heat and simmer 1 hour, stirring occasionally. Add parsnips and potatoes, if using, and cook 15 minutes more, until vegetables are tender. Add chopped tomato just before serving. Serve hot. Serves 4–6.

Fish and Seafood

Baked Fish with Tomatoes, Olives, and Fennel

1 tablespoon olive oil

1 onion, finely chopped

2 garlic cloves, minced

1 fennel bulb, green stalks and outer layers removed, sliced thin

4 plum tomatoes, chopped

¼ cup Kalamata or other black olives, pitted and chopped

1 tablespoon chopped fresh basil

1 teaspoon fresh lemon juice

Salt

Freshly ground black pepper

1 pound fresh fish fillet such as halibut, monkfish, or Chilean sea bass

Preheat oven to 425 degrees F. Lightly oil four 12" x 14" pieces of aluminum foil.

In a large skillet, heat oil over medium-low heat. Add onion, garlic, and fennel. Cook 3–5 minutes. Add tomatoes and cook, stirring occasionally, 7–8 minutes. Remove from heat and stir in olives, basil, and lemon juice. Season to taste with salt and pepper.

Pat fish dry, cut into 4 pieces, and season with salt and pepper. Place each piece on a foil square. Spoon equal amounts of sauce over each piece of fish. Form a packet of foil around each piece of fish, sealing the edges tightly so that no steam can escape.

Bake packets in oven for about 15 minutes, until fish is opaque and cooked through. Serves 4.

Rolled Fillets of Sole with Crabmeat

½ pound fresh crabmeat, picked over
1 scallion, diced
Salt
Freshly ground black pepper
1 pound of sole, cut into 4 equal portions
2 tablespoons grated cheese (Parmesan or Romano)

Preheat oven to 400 degrees F. Mix crabmeat with scallion and salt and pepper to taste. Divide crabmeat mixture equally among portions of sole and wrap each fillet around crabmeat mixture, sealing with a toothpick.

Place fillets in baking dish and sprinkle with grated cheese. Bake for 20 minutes or until fish is no longer translucent. The baking dish may be placed under the broiler for a minute or two to melt and brown the cheese before serving. Serves 2–4.

Note: The fish emits enough liquid so that you do not have to add any additional liquid. Peeled and deveined shrimp may be substituted for the crabmeat.

Broiled Scallops

1 pound scallops
1 tablespoon butter, softened
1 garlic clove, minced
½ cup chopped parsley
1 lemon, cut into wedges

Preheat broiler. In a small bowl, combine scallops, butter, garlic, and parsley. Place in a baking dish and broil for 10 minutes, stirring once.

Serve with lemon wedges. Serves 2–4.

Shrimp with Herbs

4 pounds shrimp, cooked, peeled, and deveined
2 red onions, peeled and sliced thin
2 lemons, washed and sliced thin
1 cup black olives, pitted and chopped
2 cups artichoke hearts, halved
4 tablespoons chopped pimento (optional)
½ cup olive oil
1 cup fresh lemon juice
2 tablespoons wine vinegar
1 bay leaf
Salt, to taste
Freshly ground black pepper, to taste

Combine all ingredients in a large bowl and chill. Serve cold. Serves 10.

Meats, Poultry, and Eggs

Goat Cheese and Herb Stuffed Chicken Breasts

3 whole boneless chicken breasts, skin left on
8 ounces soft goat cheese
3 tablespoons minced fresh oregano
3 tablespoons minced fresh thyme
1 tablespoon minced fresh garlic
Freshly ground black pepper
2 tablespoons olive oil
¾ cup white wine

Preheat oven to 375 degrees F. Divide the chicken breasts in half, removing the cartilage. Loosen the skin from the meat by running a finger underneath skin.

Combine goat cheese, herbs, garlic, and pepper. Place an equal portion of the cheese mixture between the skin and the meat of each breast. Replace the skin over the cheese and tuck all the edges of the skin and meat underneath each breast to form six neat packages. Arrange the breasts in a large roasting pan.

Brush the chicken breasts with olive oil. Roast for 25–35 minutes, or until the chicken is golden brown and cooked through. Remove and place on a warm platter.

Pour off the fat from the roasting pan. Place the pan over medium-high heat. Add the wine and deglaze, scraping the pan and blending bits of cheese with the wine. Serve the chicken with this sauce on the side. Serves 6.

Sautéed Calf's Liver with Onions

3 tablespoons canola or safflower oil
3 cups thinly sliced onions
Salt
Freshly ground black pepper
1½ pounds choice, pale pink calf's liver, cut into ¼" slices

In a large skillet or sauté pan, heat oil over medium-low heat. Add onion and salt and pepper to taste. Cook until onion is limp and lightly caramelized, about 20 minutes.

Using a slotted spoon or spatula, remove onion from skillet and set aside. Do not remove oil. Turn heat to high. When oil is hot, add liver, being careful not to overlap slices. (They can be sautéed in batches.) When the liver loses its raw color, turn it over and cook for 10 seconds more. Transfer to a warm plate and continue until all batches of liver are done.

Return all of the liver to the pan, add the cooked onions and stir to coat completely. Add more salt and pepper, if desired. Transfer to a warm plate and serve immediately. Serves 2–4.

Veal Chops with Wine and Mushrooms

1 teaspoon plus 3 tablespoons olive oil
½ pound fresh mushrooms, sliced
1 onion, thinly sliced
1 garlic clove, chopped fine
4 veal loin chops
1 cup red or white wine
3 tablespoons chopped parsley leaves

In a small fry pan, heat olive oil over medium heat. Add mushrooms and sauté until wilted, about 5 minutes. Set aside.

In a large sauté pan, heat 3 tablespoons olive oil over medium-high heat. Add onion and garlic and cook until onion is wilted and garlic is browned. Using a slotted spoon, remove onion slices from the pan, leaving as much garlic as possible in the pan.

In the same pan, place chops and brown on both sides, about 8–10 minutes. When chops are done, return onion to pan and add mushrooms and wine. Cook until wine is reduced by at least one half and the chops are glazed.

Sprinkle with parsley before serving. Serves 4.

Baked Chicken Roll–Ups

4 boneless, skinless chicken breasts, cut in half
16 broccoli stalks
8 carrot sticks, about ¼" thick, peeled
½ pound of muenster cheese, shredded
¼ cup chopped parsley
Olive oil spray

Preheat oven to 350 degrees F. Lay chicken breasts flat. Place two stalks of broccoli and a carrot stick on top of each piece. Roll each breast around the vegetables, allowing the broccoli floret to show at the top of the rolled chicken breast. Place the breasts side by side in a baking dish sprayed with olive oil.

Sprinkle grated cheese and parsley over the chicken. Cover with aluminum foil and bake for 20 minutes. Remove foil and bake 10 minutes more. For additional browning, place under broiler for 2–3 minutes. Drain off excess liquid before serving. Serves 4.

Pork Chops with Orange and Ginger

⅓ cup fresh orange juice
½ teaspoon freshly grated ginger
4 pork chops
1 lemon, thickly sliced

Preheat oven to 350 degrees F. In a small bowl, mix orange juice and ginger.

Place the pork chops in a baking dish and cover with the orange juice mixture. Top each chop with a slice of lemon.

Cover with aluminum foil and bake for 1 hour. To reduce the amount of liquid, you may remove the foil for the last 10 minutes of baking. Pour off excess liquid. Serves 4.

Pork Chops with Potatoes and Onions

4 pork chops
3 medium baking potatoes, peeled and sliced ½ inch thin
2 medium yellow onions, peeled and sliced thin
½ lemon, sliced thin
½ cup grated romano cheese

Place pork chops in sauté pan. Sprinkle with 2 tablespoons of romano cheese. Next layer the potatoes on top of the pork chops that have been sprinkled with cheese and sprinkle with 2 more tablespoons of romano cheese on top of the potatoes. Lastly, layer the sliced onions on top of the potatoes and chops and sprinkle with the remaining cheese. Add lemon slices around the edge of the pan. Add some water to cover the bottom of the pan to prevent scorching. Cover tightly.

Cook over medium heat for about 30–45 minutes or until chops are cooked thoroughly. The chops will flake easily with a fork. Discard the lemon slices. Serves 4.

Chicken Stir Fry

½ cup broth (chicken or vegetable)
¼ cup chopped celery
¼ cup chopped onion
1 pound boneless, skinless chicken breast, cut into thin strips
2 cups broccoli florets
1 red pepper, cut into thin strips
1 green pepper, cut into thin strips
6 pearl onions, peeled
1 cup shredded red cabbage
1 cup pea pods
¼ cup bean sprouts
¼ cup plus 2 tablespoons low-sodium soy sauce

In a large fry pan with a tight fitting cover, sauté onion and celery in broth over medium-high heat until translucent. Add chicken and 2 tablespoons soy sauce and cook until chicken is no longer pink, about 4–5 minutes.

Add vegetables and stir. Add remaining soy sauce. Cover and steam no more than five minutes. Serves 4–6.

Note: Serve over brown rice.

Stuffed Turkey Breast

1 turkey breast, boned (ask your butcher to bone it for you), about 5 pounds
Salt
Freshly ground black pepper
½ pound spicy Italian sausage, casing removed
1 tablespoon olive oil
1 pound fresh spinach or kale, rinsed thoroughly
½ cup pine nuts, lightly toasted
1 egg
¼ cup minced parsley
Pinch of oregano
1 garlic clove, peeled
¼ cup grated Parmesan cheese

½ teaspoon crushed red pepper

1 cup broth (chicken or vegetable)

Preheat oven to 350 degrees F. Pound the turkey breast flat and lightly season with salt and pepper. In a medium fry pan, cook sausage over medium heat, separating with a fork. When browned, drain the fat and remove the meat from pan. Set aside in a large bowl.

In a sauté pan, heat olive oil over medium-high heat. Add whole garlic clove and cook until browned, then discard. Add spinach or kale and sauté until wilted. Drain and wrap in cheese cloth, squeezing to remove excess moisture. Add to sausage. Add remaining ingredients, except broth, and mix to combine. Spread mixture evenly on flat turkey breast. Beginning with the long side, roll the breast around the sausage mixture. Tie with string in several places to secure.

Place rolled turkey breast in a large roasting pan with broth. Roast for about 2 hours (about 25 minutes per pound), depending on the size of the breast, basting every half hour with pan juices. When cooked through, remove from pan, cut twine, and let rest 10–15 minutes before slicing. Serves 6–8.

Note: You may substitute a large chicken breast for the turkey.

Breadless Meat Loaf

1 pound ground beef or veal, or a combination of the two

1 scallion, chopped

1 carrot, shredded

1 egg, lightly beaten

½ cup oatmeal (not instant)

½ cup fresh parsley

2 tomatoes, chopped

1 green pepper, sliced thin

Preheat oven to 350 degrees F. Combine all ingredients, except tomatoes and green pepper, in a large mixing bowl. Spread in a 9" x 5" glass loaf pan.

Cover with chopped tomatoes and slices of green pepper. Bake for 1 hour. Serves 2–4.

Off-White Egg Omelets

4 eggs, separated
1 teaspoon olive oil
Salt
Freshly ground black pepper
Optional ingredients (see below)

Separate eggs, discarding all but one yolk. Whisk together the 4 egg whites and 1 yolk with a fork.

Heat olive oil over medium heat in a nonstick pan. Add egg mixture and cook until omelet starts to form. Lift sides and let uncooked egg slide underneath until egg is cooked through. Season lightly with salt and pepper and add optional ingredients. Flip half of omelet over to cover filling ingredients. Remove from pan. Serves 1.

Optional Ingredients:
Grated Parmesan cheese and basil leaves
Fresh mozzarella cheese, basil leaves, and chopped tomato
Swiss cheese and sliced prosciutto
Swiss cheese and steamed broccoli
Fresh herbs such as sage, thyme, oregano, or rosemary
Red and green pepper slices, red onion, and tomato
Fresh salsa, mozzarella cheese, and hot sauce
Sautéed potato and onion slices
Goat cheese and fresh sage leaves
Steamed asparagus and goat cheese

Vegetables

Butternut Squash Purée with Orange and Ginger

1 medium butternut squash, peeled and seeded, cut into ½-inch cubes
1½ teaspoons grated fresh ginger
1 teaspoon grated orange rind
1 teaspoon salt, plus more to taste
Freshly ground black pepper

Steam squash in medium saucepan until tender, about 10–15 minutes. Drain excess liquid.

Place squash in the bowl of a food processor with ginger and orange rind. Process until smooth. Add salt and pepper to taste. Serve immediately. Serves 4.

Sugar Snap Peas with Arugula Pesto

2 bunches of arugula, coarse stems discarded and the leaves washed well and spun dry (about 6 packed cups)
1½ cups shelled walnuts
¾ cup freshly grated Parmesan cheese
1 teaspoon salt
1 large garlic clove, chopped
⅓ cup olive oil
1–2 pounds sugar snap peas, washed and trimmed

To make the pesto, combine the arugula, walnuts, parmesan, salt and garlic in the bowl of a food processor. Pulse until the walnuts are chopped fine. With the motor running, add oil in a stream and blend until pesto is smooth.

In a large saucepan of salted boiling water, blanch the sugar snap peas for 45 seconds, until they are crisp-tender.

Transfer peas to a large bowl and toss with enough pesto to cover generously. Serve immediately or at room temperature. Serves 4–6.

Note: Any leftover pesto will keep for 2 weeks if chilled and well covered with plastic wrap.

Roasted Winter Vegetables

6 medium beets, scrubbed, peeled, and quartered
2 medium sweet potatoes, washed and sliced into ½-inch rounds
2 red onions, outermost skin removed, quartered
20 Brussels sprouts
3 parsnips, washed and quartered lengthwise
2 baby eggplant, tops removed, quartered
¼ cup olive oil
3 sprigs fresh rosemary
3 sprigs fresh thyme
Salt
Freshly ground black pepper

Preheat oven to 425 degrees F. With a paring knife, cross-hatch the bottom of each Brussels sprout. Toss all of the vegetables together with the olive oil to coat. Toss with herbs. Season lightly with salt and pepper.

Rub excess olive oil on 2–3 baking sheets or glass baking dishes. Spread vegetables on baking sheets or dishes, place in oven, and immediately reduce oven temperature to 375 degrees F. Roast for about an hour. Some vegetables, like onions, may cook faster, so they can be removed first. Serve hot or at room temperature. Serves 6–8.

Simple Kale and Parsnips

1½ cups chicken broth (preferably homemade)
½ pound fresh parsnips, scrubbed and sliced into ½-inch rounds
1 bunch fresh kale, rinsed well and chopped
Salt
Freshly ground black pepper
Caraway seeds (optional)

Place chicken broth and sliced parsnips in a saucepan over medium heat and cook for 3–5 minutes. Add kale, and cook until kale is wilted and parsnips are soft, approximately 5 minutes more. Season with salt, pepper, and caraway seeds, if desired. Serve hot. Serves 2–4.

Braised Red Cabbage

2 tablespoons olive oil
1 head red cabbage, core removed, sliced thin
½ cup chopped onions
1 apple, peeled and cubed
¼ cup chicken broth
1 tablespoon cider vinegar
2 cloves
2 tablespoons honey (optional)

Heat olive oil over medium-high heat in a large sauté pan. Add cabbage and onion and cook until wilted.

Add apple, broth, vinegar, cloves, and honey (optional). Cover and cook 15 minutes more. Serve warm. Serves 4–6.

Spinach Pie

1 pound ricotta cheese
1 cup grated cheese (feta, mozzarella, or cheddar)
1 pound fresh spinach, cooked and drained in cheese cloth
3 eggs, lightly beaten
2 tablespoons olive oil
Optional ingredients: ½ cup sliced and sautéed zucchini, *or* 1 cup diced red or green pepper
Salt
Freshly ground black pepper
½ cup chopped, cooked meat such as ham or bacon
½ cup fresh mushrooms

Preheat oven to 350 degrees F. Combine ricotta, grated cheese, spinach, eggs, and 1 tablespoon olive oil in a blender or food processor. Mix until blended. Add optional ingredients at this time, and stir by hand to combine. Season with salt and pepper to taste.

Pour into a 10" glass pie plate that has been rubbed with additional olive oil. Drizzle remaining olive oil over the top. Bake for about 45 minutes or until a knife inserted in the center comes out clean. The top will be browned. Allow to cool slightly before cutting. Serves 6–8.

Dessert

Baked Custard

2 cups skim milk
½ teaspoon vanilla extract
4 eggs
Cinnamon

Preheat oven to 325 degrees F. In a small saucepan, heat milk to a simmer over medium heat. In a mixing bowl, beat eggs. Slowly pour hot milk into beaten eggs and whisk to combine. Stir in the vanilla. Strain into 4 or 5 custard cups set in a large baking pan. Add water to the pan until it comes halfway up the side of each cup. Lightly sprinkle cinnamon over the top of each custard.

Bake custards for 1 hour or until a knife inserted in the middle comes out clean. Chill thoroughly and serve with fresh fruit. Serves 4 or 5.

Bibliography

Chapter One

Alfthan, G., A. Aro and K.F. Gey. "Plasma homocysteine and cardiovascular disease mortality." *Lancet* (1997) 349:397.

Ellis, J.M. and K.S. McCully. "Prevention of myocardial infarction by vitamin B6." *Research Communications in Molecular Pathology and Pharmacology* (1995) 89:208–220.

Graham, I.H., H.M. Refsum, I.H. Rosenberg, and P.M. Ueland. *Homocysteine Metabolism: From Basic Science to Clinical Medicine.* Boston: Kluwer, 1997.

Graham, I.H. "Plasma homocysteine as a risk factor for vascular disease. The European concerted action project." *Journal of the American Medical Association* (1997) 277:1775–1781.

Havlik, R.J. and M. Feinleib, eds. *Proceedings of the Conference on Decline in Coronary Heart Disease Mortality.* Bethesda: NIH Publication No. 79–1610, 1979.

Keys, A. "Coronary heart disease: The global picture." *Atherosclerosis* (1975) 22:149–192.

Malinow, M.R., P.B. Duell, D.L. Hess, P.H. Anderson, W.D. Kruger, B.E. Phillipson, R.A. Gluckman, P.C. Block, and B.M. Upson. "Reduction of plasmahomocysteine levels by breakfast cereal fortified with folic acid in patients with coronary heart disease." *New England Journal of Medicine* (1998) 338:1009–1015.

McCully, K.S. *The Homocysteine Revolution: Medicine for the New Millennium.* New Canaan, CT: Keats Publishing, 1997.

McCully, K.S. "Homocysteine theory of arteriosclerosis: Development and current status." In A.M. Gotto, Jr., and R. Paoletti, eds, *Atherosclerosis Reviews*, Volume 11, New York: Raven, 1983, pp. 157–245.

McCully, K.S. "Chemical pathology of homocysteine. I Atherogenesis. II Carcinogenesis and homocysteine thiolactone metabolism. III Cellular function and aging." *Annals of Clinical and Laboratory Science* (1993) 23:477–493; (1994) 24:27–59; 134–152.

McCully, K.S. "Atherosclerosis, serum cholesterol and the homocysteine theory: A study of 194 consecutive autopsies." *American Journal of the Medical Sciences* (1990) 299:217–221.

Morrison, H.I., D. Schaubel, M. Desmeules, and D.T. Wigle. "Serum folate and risk of fatal coronary heart disease." *Journal of the American Medical Association* (1996) 275:1893–1896.

Mudd, S.H., F. Skovby, H.L. Levy, K.D. Pettigrew, B. Wilcken, R.E. Pyeritz, G. Andria, G.H.J. Boers, I.L. Bromberg, R. Cerone, B. Fowler, H. Grobe, H. Schmidt, and L. Schweitzer. "The natural history of homocystinuria due to cystathionine beta synthase deficiency." *American Journal of Human Genetics* (1985) 37:1–31.

Nygard, O., S.E. Vollset, H.M. Refsum, I. Stensvold, A. Tverdal, J.E. Nordrehaug, P.M. Ueland, and G. Kvale. "Total plasma homocysteine and cardiovascular risk profile: The Hordaland homocysteine study." *Journal of the American Medical Association* (1995) 274:1526–1533.

Nygard, O., J.E. Nordrehaug, H.M. Refsum, P.M. Ueland, M. Farstad, and S.E. Vollset. "Plasma homocysteine levels and mortality in patients with coronary artery disease." *New England Journal of Medicine* (1997) 337:230–236.

Petersen, J.C. and J.D. Spence. "Vitamins and progression of atherosclerosis in hyperhomocysteinemia." *Lancet* (1998) 351:263.

Rath, M. and A. Hiedzwiecki. "Nutritional supplement program halts progression of early coronary atherosclerosis documented by ultrafast
computed tomography." *Journal of Applied Nutrition* (1996) 48: 67–78.

Rimm, E.B., W.C. Willett, F.B. Hu, L. Sampson, G.A. Colditz, J.E.
Manson, C. Hennekens, and M.J. Stampfer. "Folate and vitamin B6
from diet and supplements in relation to risk of coronary heart disease among women." *Journal of the American Medical Association*
(1998) 279:359–364.

Selhub, J., P.F. Jacques, P.W.F. Wilson, D. Rush, and I.H. Rosenberg.
"Vitamin status and intake as primary determinants of homocys-
teinemia in an elderly population." *Journal of the American Medical
Association* (1993) 270:2693–2698.

Stampfer, M.J., M.R. Malinow, W.C. Willett, L.M. Newcomer, B. Upson,
D. Ullmann, P.V. Tishler, and C.H. Hennekens. "A prospective
study of plasma homocysteine and risk of myocardial infarction in
US physicians." *Journal of the American Medical Association* (1992)
268:877–881.

Stampfer, M.J., C.H. Hennekens, J.E. Manson, G.A. Colditz, B. Rosner,
and W.C. Willett. "Vitamin E consumption and the risk of coronary disease in women." *New England Journal of Medicine* (1993)
328:1444–1449.

Wald, N.J., Watt, H.C., Law, M.R., Weir, D.G., McPartlin, J. and Scott,
J.M. "Homocysteine and ischemic heart disease. Results of a
prospective study with implications regarding prevention."
Archives of Internal Medicine (1998)158:862–867.

Chapter Two

Beckels, G.L.A., B.R. Kirkwood, and D.C. Carson. "High total and cardiovascular disease mortality in adults of Indian descent in
Trinidad, unexplained by major risk factors." *Lancet* (1986) 1298.

Cleave, T.L. *The Saccharine Disease*. Bristol, CT: Wright, 1974.

Dietary Guidelines Advisory Committee. *Report of the Dietary Guidelines
Committee on the Dietary Guidelines for Americans*, 1995. Washington, D.C.: U.S. Department of Agriculture, 1995.

Eaton, S.B., M. Shostak, and M. Konner. *The Paleolithic Prescription*. New York: Harper & Row, 1988.

Gilman, M.W., L.A. Cupples, B.E. Millen, R.C. Ellison, and P.A. Wolf. "Inverse association of dietary fat with development of ischemic stroke in men." *New England Journal of Medicine* (1997) 278:2145–2150.

Hu, F.B., M.J. Stampfer, J.E. Manson, E. Rimm, G.A. Colditz, B.A. Rosner, C.H. Hennekens, and W.C. Willett. "Dietary fat intake and the risk of coronary heart disease in women." *New England Journal of Medicine* (1997) 337:1491–1499.

Jacobson, M.S. "Cholesterol oxides in Indian ghee: possible cause of unexplained high risk of atherosclerosis in Indian immigrant populations." *Lancet* (1987) ii:656.

Lutz, W. *Dismantling a Myth: The Role of Fat and Carbohydrates in Our Diet*. Munich: Selecta-Verlag, 1986.

McGovern, G. "Eating in America: Dietary Goals for the United States." *Report of the Select Committee on Nutrition and Human Needs*, U.S. Senate. Cambridge, MA: MIT Press, 1977.

National Research Council. *Recommended Dietary Allowances*, Eleventh Edition. Washington, D.C.: National Academy of Sciences, 1998.

Peng, S-K., and R.J. Morin. *Biological Effects of Cholesterol Oxides*. Boca Raton, FL: CRC Press, 1992.

Price, W.A. *Nutrition and Physical Degeneration*. 50th Anniversary Edition. New Canaan, CT: Keats Publishing, 1989.

Welsh, S.O., C. Davis, and A. Shaw. "A brief history of food guides in the United States." *Nutrition Today* Nov/Dec: 6–11, 1992.

Welsh, S.O., C. Davis, and A. Shaw. "USDA's Food Guide: Background and development." Washington, D.C.: United States Department of Agriculture, Publication Number 1514, 1993.

Willett, W.C. "Diet and health: What should we eat?" *Science* (1994) 264:532–537.

Chapter Three

Bauernfeind, J.C. and P.A. Lachance. *Nutrient Additions to Food. Nutritional, Technological and Regulatory Aspects*. Trumbull, CT: Food and Nutrition Press, 1991.

Fennema, O.R. *Food Chemistry*, 3d Ed. New York: Marcel Dekker, 1996.

Bibliography 215

Karmas, E. and R.S. Harris. *Nutritional Evaluation of Food Processing,* 3d Ed. New York: Van Nostrand Reinhold, 1987.

Schroeder, H.A. "Losses of vitamins and trace minerals resulting from processing and preservation of foods." *American Journal of Clinical Nutrition* (1971) 24:562–573.

Shils, M.E., Olson, J.A. and Shike, M. *Modern Nutrition in Health and Disease,* 8th Ed. Philadelphia: Lea & Febiger, 1994.

Chapter Four

Atkins, R.C. *Dr. Atkins' Diet Revolution.* New York: Bantam, 1972.

Eades, M.R. and M.D. Eades. *Protein Power.* New York: Bantam, 1996.

Eaton, S.B., M. Shostak, and M. Konner. *The Paleolithic Prescription.* New York: Harper & Row, 1988.

Lutz, W. *Dismantling a Myth. The Role of Fats and Carbohydrates in Our Diet.* Munich: Selecta-Verlag, 1986.

McCully, K.S. *The Homocysteine Revolution: Medicine for the New Millennium.* New Canaan, CT: Keats Publishing, 1997.

National Research Council. *Recommended Dietary Allowances,* 11th Edition. Washington, D.C.: National Academy of Sciences, 1998.

Sears, B. and W. Lawren. *The Zone: A Dietary Road Map.* New York: HarperCollins, 1996.

Simopoulos, A.P. and J. Robinson. *The Omega Plan.* New York: HarperCollins, 1998.

Steward, H.L., M.C. Bethea, S.S. Andrews, and L.A. Balart. *Sugar Busters.* Metairie, LA: Sugar Busters Press, 1995.

Tarnower, H. and S.S. Baker. *The Complete Scarsdale Medical Diet.* New York: Rawson Wade, 1978.

Chapter Five

Bauernfeind, J.C. and P.A. LaChance. *Nutrient Additions to Foods: Nutritional, Technological and Regulatory Aspects.* Trumbull, CT: Food & Nutrition Press, 1991.

Ellis, J.M. and K.S. McCully. "Prevention of myocardial infarction by vitamin B6." *Research Communications in Molecular Pathology and Pharmacology,* 89:208–220, 1995.

Havlik, R.J. and M. Feinleib, eds. *Proceedings of the Conference on Decline in Coronary Heart Disease Mortality.* Bethesda, MD: NIH Publication No. 79–1610, 1979.

McCully, K.S. "Homocysteine theory of arteriosclerosis: Development and current status." In R. Paoletti and A.M. Gotto, Jr. *Atherosclerosis Reviews*, Volume 11. New York: Raven Press, 1983, pp 157–246.

Morrison, H.I., D. Schaubel, M. Desmeules, and D.T. Wigle. "Serum Folate and risk of fatal coronary heart disease." *Journal of the American Medical Association* (1996) 275:1893–1896, .

National Research Council, *Recommended Dietary Allowances*, 11th Ed. Washington, D.C.: National Academy of Science, 1998.

Rimm, E.B., W.C. Willett, F.B. Hu, L. Sampson, G.A. Colditz, J.E. Manson, C. Hennekens, and M.J. Stampfer. "Folate and vitamin B6 from diet and supplements in relation to risk of coronary heart disease among women." *Journal of the American Medical Association* (1998) 279:359–333364.

Ubbink, J.B., W.J.H. Vermaak, A. VanderMerwe, P.J. Becker, R. Delport, and H.C. Potgeiter. "Vitamin requirements for the treatment of hyperhomocysteinemia in humans." *Journal of Nutrition* (1994) 124:1927–1933.

Chapter Six

Cravo, M.L., L.M. Gloria, J. Selhub, M.R. Nadeau, M.E. Camilo, M.P. Resende, J.N. Cardoso, C.N. Leitao, and F.C. Mira. "Hyperhomocysteinemia in chronic alcoholism: correlation with folate, vitamin B12 and vitamin B6 status." *American Journal of Clinical Nutrition* (1996) 63:220–224.

Fennema, O.R. *Food Chemistry*, 3d Ed. New York: Marcel Dekker, 1996.

Fox, N. *Spoiled: Why Our Foods Are Making Us Sick and What We Can Do About It.* New York: Penguin, 1998.

Goldberg, D.M. "Does wine work?" *Clinical Chemistry* (1995) 41:14–16.

Grobstein, C. and J. Cairns. *Diet, Nutrition and Cancer.* Washington, D.C.: National Academy Press, 1982.

Newman, T.B. and S.B. Hulley. "Carcinogenicity of lipid-lowering drugs." *Journal of the American Medical Association* (1996) 275:55–60.

Nygard, O., H. Refsum, P.M. Ueland, I. Stensvold, J.E. Nordrehaug, G.

Kvale, and S.E. Vollset. "Coffee consumption and plasma total homocysteine: the Hordaland Homocysteine Study." *American Journal of Clinical Nutrition* (1996) 63:136–143.

Ono, H., A. Sakamoto, T. Eguchi, N. Fujita, S. Nomura, H. Ueda, N. Sakura, and K. Ueda. "Plasma total homocysteine concentrations in epileptic patients taking anticonvulsants." *Metabolism* (1997) 46:9959–962.

Sinatra, S.T. *The Coenzyme Q10 Phenomenon* New Canaan, CT: Keats, 1998.

Ueland, P.M. and H.M. Refsum. "Plasma homocysteine, a risk factor for vascular disease: plasma levels in health, disease and drug therapy." *Journal of Clinical and Laboratory Medicine* (1989) 114:473–501.

VanderMooren, M.J., M.G.A.J. Wonters, H.J.Blom, L.A. Schellekens, T.K.A.B. Estes, and R. Rolland. "Hormone replacement therapy may reduce high serum homocysteine in postmenopausal women." *European Journal of Clinical Investigation* (1994) 24:733–736.

Chapter Seven

Anand, R.S. and P. Peter Basiotis. "Is Total Fat Consumption Really Decreasing?" *Nutrition Insights,* A Publication of the USDA Center for Nutrition Policy and Promotion, April, 1998.

Barinaga, Marcia, "How Much pain for cardiac gain." *Science*, Vol. 276, May 30, 1997.

Blair, S.N., J.C. Connelly, "How much physical actiivty should we do? The case for moderate amounts and intensities of physical activity." *Research Quarterly* (1996) 67:193–205.

Blair, S.N., H.W. Kohl III, C.E. Barlow, R.S. Paffenbarger, Jr., L.W. Gibbons, C.A. Macera. "Changes in physical fitness and all-cause mortalilty: a prospective study of healthy and unhealthy men." *Journal of the American Medical Association* (1995) 273:1093–1098.

Blair, S.N., H.W. Kohl, N.F. Gordon. "How much physical activity is good for health?" *Annual Reviews of Public Health* (1992) 13:99–126.

Dietz, W.H. "Health Consequences of Obesity in Youth: Childhood Predictors of Adult Disease." *Pediatrics* (1998).

Dunne, Lavon J., *Nutrition Almanac*. Nutrition Search, Inc. New York: McGraw-Hill, 1990.

Gortmaker, S.L., A. Must, J.M. Perrin, A.M. Sobol, W.H. Dietz. "Social and economic consequences of overweight in adolescence and young adulthood." *New England Journal of Medicine* (1993) 329:1008–12.

Kuczmarski et al., "Increasing Prevalence of Overweight Among US Adults: The National Health and Nutrition Examination Surveys, 1960 to 1991." *Journal of the American Medical Association* (1994) 272:205–211.

Lee, I.M., C.C. Hsieh, and R.S. Paffenbarger. "Exercise intensity and longevity in men: the Harvard Alumni Health Study." *Journal of the American Medical Association* (1995) 273:1179–1184.

Manson, J.E., and I.M. Lee. "Exercise for women—how much pain for optimal gain." Editorial, *New England Journal of Medicine* (1996) 334:1325–7.

Manson, J.E., W.C. Willett, M.J. Stampfer, G.A. Colditz, D.J. Hunter, S.E. Hankinson et al. "Body weight and mortality among women." *New England Journal of Medicine* (1995) 333:677–685.

Munoz, K.A., S.M. Krebs-Smith, R. Ballard-Barbash, and L.E. Cleveland, "Food intakes of US children and adolescents compared with recommendations." *Pediatrics* (1997) 100:323–329.

Nygard, Ottar MD et al., "total plasma homocysteine and cardiovascular risk profile: The Hordaland homocysteine study." *Journal of the American Medical Association* (1995) 274: 1526–33.

Paffenbarger, R.S., Jr, R.T. Hyde, A.L. Wing, I.M. Lee, D.L. Jung, J.B. Kampert. "The association of changes in physical activity level and other lifestyle characteristics with mortality among men." *New England Journal of Medicine* (1993) 328:538–545.

Pate, R.R., M Pratt, S.N. Blair et al. "Physical Activity and Public Health: A Recommendation from the Centers for Disease Control and Prevention and the American College of Sports Medicine." *Journal of the American Medical Association* (1995) 273:402–407.

U.S. Department of Health and Human Services. "Update: Prevalence of Overweight Among Children, Adolescents, and Adults—United States 1988–1994." *Mortality and Morbidity Weekly Report*, Vol. 46. No. 9.

U.S. Department of Health and Human Services. *Physical Activity and Health: A Report of the Surgeon General*. Atlanta, GA: U.S. Department of Health and Human Services, Centers for Disease Control and Prevention, National Center for Chronic Disease Prevention and Health Promotion, 1996.

U.S. Department of Health and Human Services, Centers for Disease Control and Prevention. "Public health focus: physical activity and the prevention of cornonary heart disease." *Mortality and Morbidity Weekly Report* (1993) 42 (35):669–672.

Williams, P.T. "Relationship of distance run per week to coronary heart disease risk factors in 8283 male runners." *Archive of Internal Medicine* (1997);157–191–198.

Chapter Eight

Dilman, V. and W. Dean. *The Neuroendocrine Theory of Aging and Degenerative Disease*. Pensacola, FL: The Center for Bio-Gerontology, 1992.

Finch, C.E. *Longevity, Senescence and the Genome*. Chicago: University of Chicago Press, 1990.

Harman, D. "Aging: A theory based on free radical and radiation chemistry." *Journal of Gerontology* (1956) 11:298–300.

Hayflick, L. "The limited in vitro lifetime of human diploid cell strains." *Experimental Cell Research* (1965) 37:614–636.

McCully, K.S. "Chemical pathology of homocysteine. III Cellular function and aging." *Annals of Clinical and Laboratory Science* (1994) 24:134–152.

McCully, K.S. *The Homocysteine Revolution: Medicine for the New Millennium*. New Canaan, CT: Keats Publishing, 1997.

Olszewski, A.J., W.B. Szostak, M. Bialkowska, S. Rudnicki, and K.S. McCully. "Reduction of plasma lipid and homocysteine levels by pyridoxine, folate, cobalamin, choline, riboflavin and troxerutin in atherosclerosis." *Atherosclerosis* (1989) 75:1–9.

Sinatra, S.T. *The Coenzyme Q10 Phenomenon*. New Canaan, CT: Keats Publishing, 1998.

Yudkin, J. and S. Stanner. *Eating for a Healthy Heart*. New Canaan, CT: Keats Publishing, 1997.

Chapter Nine

Clarke, R., A.D. Smith, K.A. Jobst, H. Refsum, L. Sutton, and P.M. Ueland. "Folate, vitamin B12, and serum total homocysteine levels in confirmed Alzheimer's disease." *Archives of Neurology* (1998) 55:1449–1455.

Grant, W.B. "Eating more fish and less fat results in a lower incidence of Alzheimer's disease." *Nutritional Therapy Today* (1998) 8:8–9.

Jackson, L.A., L.A. Campbell, R.A. Schmidt, C-C. Kuo, A.L. Cappuccio, M.J. Lee, and J.T. Grayston, "Specificity of detection of Chlamydia pneumoniae in cardiovascular atheroma. Evaluation of the innocent bystander hypothesis." *American Journal of Pathology* (1997) 150:1785–1790.

Lipton, S.A., W-K. Kim, Y-B. Choi, S. Kumar, D.M. D'Emilia, P.V. Rayudu, D.R. Arnelle, and J.S. Stamler "Neurotoxicity associated with dual actions of homocysteine at the N-methyl-D-aspartate receptor." *Proceedings of the National Academy of Sciences USA* (1997) 94:5923–5928.

Petrie, M., R. Roubenoff, G.E. Dallal, , M.R. Nadeau, J. Selhub, and I.H. Rosenberg. "Plasma homocysteine as a risk factor for atherothrombotic events in systemic lupus erythematosus." *Lancet* (1996) 348:1120–1124.

Quinn, C.T., J.C. Griener, T. Bottiglieri, K. Hyland, A. Farrow, and B.A. Kamen. "Elevation of homocysteine and excitatory amino acid neurotransmitters in the CSF of children who receive methotrexate for the treatment of cancer." *Journal of Clinical Oncology* (1997) 15:2800–2806.

Regland, B., M. Andersson, L. Abrahamsson, L.E. Dyrehag, and C.G. Gottfries. "Increased concentrations of homocysteine in the cerebrospinal fluid in patients with fibromyalgia and chronic fatigue syndrome." *Scandinavian Journal of Rheumatology* (1997) 26:301–307.

Regland, B., B.V. Johansson, B. Grenfeldt, L.T. Hjelmgren, and M. Medhus. "Homocysteinemia is a common feature of schizophrenia." *Journal of Neural Transmission* (1995) 100:165–169.

Riggs, K.M., A. Spiro, K.Tucker, and D. Rush, "Relations of vitamin B12, vitamin B6, folate and homocysteine to cognitive performance in the Normative Aging Study." *American Journal of Clinical Nutrition* (1996) 63:306–314.

Roubenoff, R., P. Dellaripa, M.R. Nadeau, L.W. Abad, B.A. Muldoon, J. Selhub, and I.H. Rosenberg. "Abnormal homocysteine metabolism in rheumatoid arthritis." *Arthritis and Rheumatism* (1997) 40:718–722.

Santhosh-Kumar, C.R., K.L. Hassell, J.C. Deutsch, and J.F. Kolhouse. "Are neuropsychiatric manifestations of folate, cobalamin and pyridoxine deficiency mediated through imbalances in excitatory sulfur amino acids?" *Medical Hypotheses* (1994) 43:239–244.

Sauberlich, H.E. "Relationship of vitamin B6, vitamin B12, and folate to neurological and neuropsychiatric disorders." In A. Bendich and C.E. Butterworth, Jr., eds., *Micronutrients in Health and in Disease Prevention*. New York: Marcel Dekker, 1991, pp 187–218.

Sung, J.J.Y. and J.E. Sanderson. "Hyperhomocysteinemia, Helicobacter pylori, and coronary heart disease." *Heart* (1996) 76:305–307.

Index

Arteriosclerosis (*cont.*)
  smoking and, 133–34
  vegetarianism and, 12, 81
  vitamin B6 deficiency and, 9–10,
    11, 105
  vitamin supplements and, 114
Arugula pesto, snap peas with, 206
Atherosclerosis, 28
Autoimmune disease, 185–86
Azaribine, 128–29

Bacon, 121
Bagels, 38, 48
Baked custard, 209
Baked fish with tomatoes, olives,
    and fennel, 197–98
Baked goods, 48
Baking, 94
Beans, vegetable soup with, 196–97
Beer, 133, 140
Beets, wheatberry salad with, 191–92
Beriberi, 51
Beta-carotene, 165–66
Betaine, 172, 173
Bilirubin, 161
Bioflavonoids, 165
Birth control pills, 136–37, 140
Bleaching agents, 58
Blood cholesterol levels
  dietary cholesterol and, 14–15, 17,
    19
  heart disease and, 19
Blood clot, 28
Blood homocysteine levels
  arteriosclerosis and, 9–10
  cholesterol-lowering drugs and, 20
  drugs and, 11, 127–29
  factors increasing levels of, 11
  heart disease and, 23–24
  Heart Revolution diet and lower-
    ing of, 5
  homocystinuria and, 7–9
  hormones and, 135–38
  low-density lipoprotein (LDL)
    and, 16, 20

vitamin B6, vitamin B12, and folic
    acid and, 9–10, 15–16, 18, 22
Blood pressure
  carbohydrates and, 46
  heart attack risk and, 24
  Heart Revolution diet and lower-
    ing of, 5
  homocysteine levels and, 11
  See also Hypertension
Blood tests, for homocysteine, 114,
    116
Borscht, 196
Brain
  homocysteine and, 179–80
  vitamin deficiencies and,
    180–83
Braised red cabbage, 207
Breadless meat loaf, 204
Breads, 38, 48, 68, 69, 170
Breakfast
  Heart Revolution diet and, 91
  menu suggestions for, 97–101
Broiled scallops, 198
Brown rice, 41, 60, 101, 193
Bulk minerals, 67
Butter, 70, 85
  processing of, 43–44, 48
Butternut squash puree with orange
    and ginger, 205
B vitamin deficiencies
  food guidelines and, 46–47
  heart disease and, 2, 12, 107–8
  processed food and, 12, 14
B vitamins
  aging and need for, 73–74, 75–76
  Alzheimer's disease and, 176
  blood homocysteine levels, 9–10,
    15–16
  food processing and loss of, 42
  health and key role of, 26–27
  See also Folic acid; Vitamin B6;
    Vitamin B12
B vitamin supplements
  arteriosclerosis prevention and, 26
  Heart Revolution diet with, 5

Quercetin, 165
Quinoa salad, 192–93

Recipes
  dessert, 209
  fish and seafood, 197–99
  hors-d'oeuvres, 193–95
  meat, poultry, and eggs, 199–205
  salads, 191–93
  soups, 195–97
  vegetables, 205–8
Recommended Dietary Allowance
  (RDA), 34, 35, 47, 188–89
Red cabbage, 207
Red dye #2, 120
Red wine, 132, 140, 165, 169
Refined carbohydrates, 40, 46, 47,
  78
Restaurant food, 95–96
Retinoids, 164
Rheumatoid arthritis, 185, 186
Riboflavin, 64
Rice, 48
  Food Pyramid on, 38
  refining of, 40, 41, 60, 61
  vitamin B1 deficiency and, 51
Rickets, 51, 104
Rinehart, James, 9–10
Roasted nuts, 193–94
Roasted winter vegetables,
  206–7
Rolled filets of sole with crabmeat,
  198
Roll ups, baked chicken, 201

Salad dressing, 70
Salads
  Heart Revolution diet and, 92
  recipes for, 191–93
Saturated fat, 44
Sautéed calf's liver with onions,
  200
Scallops, 198
Schizophrenia, 181
Scurvy, 51

Seafood, recipes for, 197–99
Selenium, 67, 173, 174
Shopping for food, 124–26, 139
Shrimp with herbs, 199
Simvistatin, 129
Skim milk, 70
Smoked foods, 104, 122–23, 139,
  167
Smoking
  free radicals in, 166–67
  health and, 133–34, 140
  heart attack risk and, 24
Snacks, 102
  menu suggestions for, 97–101
Snap peas with arugula pesto, 206
Sodium, 67
Sole with crabmeat, 198
Soups, recipes for, 195–97
Spinach pie, 208
Spreads
  chicken liver, 194
  white bean, 195
Statin drugs, 19–20, 129–31, 139,
  164
Sterilization, in food processing, 56,
  62, 104
Stir-fry, chicken, 202–3
Strength training, 151–52, 155
Stretching, 152, 155
Stroke
  definition of, 30
  exercise and, 147, 149
  fat intake and, 46, 83
  hemorrhagic. See Hemorrhagic
    stroke
Stuffed turkey breast, 203–4
Sucrose, 55
Sugar, 40, 41–42, 54–55, 70
Sugar snap peas with arugula pesto,
  206
Sulfate, 64, 161
Supplements. See Food fortification;
  Vitamin supplements
Synthetic foods, 123–24
Szent-Gyorgi, Albert, 10